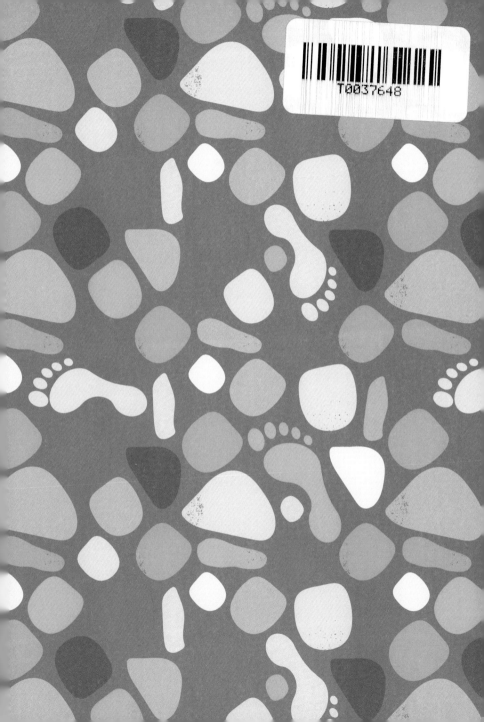

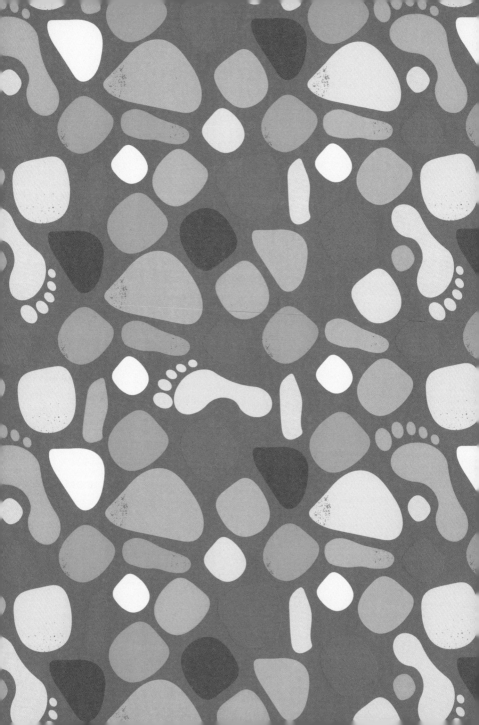

· THE ·
FOOT
BOOK

THE CARE AND KEEPING
· OF YOUR FEET ·

DR. TODD BRENNAN,
DPM, FACFAS, FABPM
OF HEALTHY FEET PODIATRY

&

DR. LESLIE JOHNSTON, DPM

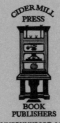

CIDER MILL
PRESS

BOOK
PUBLISHERS
KENNEBUNKPORT, MAINE

CONTENTS

INTRODUCTION

What's wrong with my feet? Type this question into Google, and you'll get a million responses. You can ask a general doctor what's wrong with your feet, and he or she will usually say, "I don't know." You would be surprised how little the medical community really knows about foot problems. That's why most primary care doctors have a podiatrist in their toolbox of referral sources.

So why write a general medical book about feet? The simple answer is this: to educate the general public and our medical community about what podiatrists do. The field of podiatry has evolved since the earlier careers of our colleagues, and because podiatry has not remained a stagnant profession, many people don't know what we do!

Early on in our careers, my wife and I used to get irritated, and even angry at times, because we went through the years of schooling, and then the rigorous training in residency, and when the time came to start a "real" job, we were confronted with the harsh reality that most of the medical community (medical doctors, nurses, chiropractors, etc.) thought we trimmed toenails all day. Now don't get us wrong; we trim nails. But there is so much more to our field of study. New subspecialties have emerged that podiatrists have become passionate about learning and improving. Surgery, wound care, and biomechanics are just a few examples of the subspecialties in our profession.

So as time moved on and we developed closer relationships with other medical professionals, we began to realize the importance of educating everyone about the career about which we are passionate: podiatry. Medical doctors didn't know what we did, not because they thought our career was unimportant, but because they had no reference as to what we currently are trained to do. The same statement goes for the general public as well. So we thought writing *The Foot Book* would be a great way not only to discuss foot problems, but also educate the general public and medical community on what a podiatrist does.

We've gathered our knowledge from over twenty years of combined experience and generated a layman's book about foot problems and how to treat them. This book was written for you to understand the most common foot problems that we, as podiatrists, diagnose and treat in our offices. We will admit it has been difficult to explain some of the complexities of the foot in terms the general public can easily understand; however, after the completion of the book, we feel that you or your primary care doctor can read this and learn something important.

I hope *The Foot Book* will be an excellent resource for home libraries and waiting rooms. And I hope that you not only learn something about your feet but about podiatry as well.

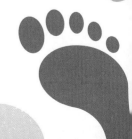

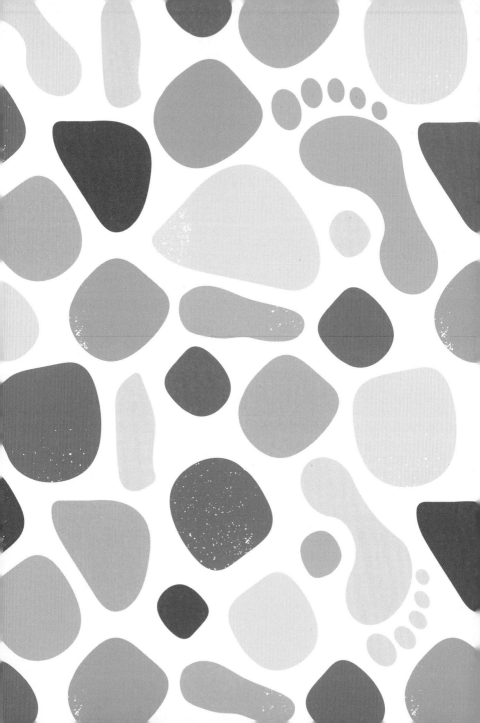

CHAPTER 1

TAKING CARE OF YOUR FEET

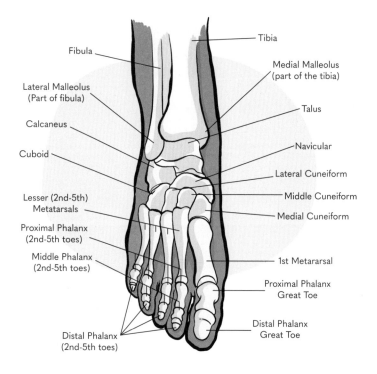

Tibia

Fibula

Medial Malleolus
(part of the tibia)

Lateral Malleolus
(Part of fibula)

Talus

Calcaneus

Cuboid

Navicular

Lateral Cuneiform

Lesser (2nd-5th)
Metatarsals

Middle Cuneiform

Medial Cuneiform

Proximal Phalanx
(2nd-5th toes)

Middle Phalanx
(2nd-5th toes)

1st Metararsal

Proximal Phalanx
Great Toe

Distal Phalanx
Great Toe

Distal Phalanx
(2nd-5th toes)

The foot: the foundation of your body. It is complex, yet engineered with the simplicity of the levers of physics. A functional marvel that allows our bodies to run marathons, stand in line at the amusement park for hours, and perform the simple task of putting one foot in front of the other. The foot is composed of 26 bones and 33 joints. Your feet comprise one-quarter of all the bones in your body. With over a hundred soft tissue structures, including tendons and ligaments, every movement has a purpose—to provide mobility. With that said, many people neglect their feet until they can't walk. If you sustain an injury to your eye or have a cavity in your tooth, you typically go to the optometrist or dentist right away to get it fixed. But if your feet hurt, rather than find your local podiatrist, you try home remedies or use infomercial products with a Hail Mary in hopes that your foot pain will magically go away. Why is that? Most people are not fully aware of what podiatrists are or what we can do for your feet.

In this book, I'll examine common foot problems, treatments you can do at home, and treatments your podiatrist can do as well. I'll also discuss some common misunderstandings or misconceptions associated with foot conditions, such as heel spurs, ingrown toenails, and bunions, just to name a few.

Let's start with the most obvious ways you can help your feet: take care of your body and be mindful of your diet. The more you eat, the more weight you'll gain. The more weight you gain, the more pressure and stress your feet are under, increasing the risk of foot problems. If you are overweight, there is a higher probability that your feet are going to hurt. While it is possible to be pain-free and overweight, there is a higher likelihood for recurrence of pain when more stress is placed on the foot.

What other conditions can indirectly affect your foot, besides obesity? Cigarette smoking, abuse of alcohol, and poor diet can contribute to foot problems. Poor blood flow caused by plaque buildup in your arteries can dramatically affect the tiny blood vessels all the way down to your toes, increasing the risk for nonhealing wounds on your feet. Decreased blood flow leads to increased pain with rest or walking and higher risk of tissue damage, tissue loss, or necrosis. These sound like extreme issues; however, these conditions tend to manifest as we get older. The harder we are on our bodies physically when we're younger, or the more we neglect the nutritional needs our bodies crave, the more likely it is that later on in life, we will come face to face with the repercussions of our earlier decisions.

It would be unrealistic of me to tell you not to walk barefoot and always wear shoes; however, assuring that you have proper support on your feet is imperative in the long term to help prevent foot problems. Moderation is always key. Knowing when to wear supportive shoes and leave the flip-flops at home will give you the opportunity to make the better choice in your shoe gear. As a realist, I understand that my patients are going to go barefoot from time to time, especially since I practice in Florida. We will address shoe selection in the next chapter, but ensuring the regular use of supportive, quality shoes and orthotics is important for reducing your risk of foot problems.

If you work out or are generally an active person, stretching exercises for your feet before and after workouts are helpful to reduce the risk of injury to your feet and ankles. Warming up the body and performing light stretching prior to a more rigorous workout will decrease the risk of a muscle strain, tendon tear, or ligament sprain. Proper cooldowns after a workout and appropriate stretching also help decrease the risk of injury to the foot and ankle. Stretching exercises such as heel cord stretches (straight leg, knee bent), towel calf stretches, and ankle joint range-of-motion exercises are just a

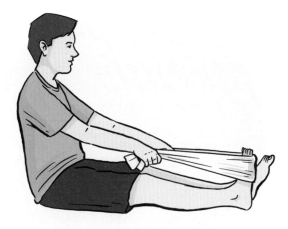

Towel calf stretch

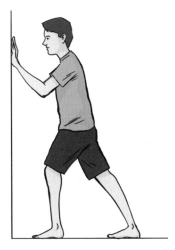

Heel cord stretch straight leg

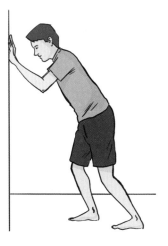

Heel cord stretch knee bent

few of the simple warm-ups for the foot and ankle that can be incorporated prior to starting your activity or workout.

DAILY FOOT CHECKS. Whether you are diabetic or not, you should check your feet on a regular basis. What are you looking for? Any unfamiliar moles on the bottom of your foot or between your toes could be a potential skin cancer and should be checked out. Any dark discoloration under your nail without a known reason? Again, this should be checked by a podiatrist for an unknown injury to the nail plate or a rare skin cancer as well. These are just a few examples of things to look for during a routine foot check.

As we progress through the book, there will be more pathologies you can look for at home and know whether or not you should see a podiatrist. If you make it a point to check your feet regularly before or after showering, that will make it easier to remember, and it will become a part of your routine. Knowing how your foot feels or looks normally will help when you do find a new problem over time.

Be proactive in your foot health. A lot of foot problems are hereditary or genetic. If you know your parents or grandparents have a history of foot problems and/or surgery, understand why it occurred and how to prevent it from happening to you as well. Once you get an accurate family history, check in with a podiatrist to formulate a plan.

DEFINITIONS OF COMMONLY USED TERMS WITH REGARD TO FEET AND ANKLES

Ankle Joint: The main joint that connects the leg to the foot

Bilateral: Occurring on both sides of the body

Distal: Furthest distance from the main mass of the body

Dorsal: The top of the foot

Dorsiflexion: Movement of a joint in an upward position

Eversion: Movement of a joint away from the midline of the body

Frontal Plane: Separates the body into front and back halves

Interphalangeal Joint (IPJ): The small joints in the toes

Inversion: Movement of a joint toward the midline of the body

Lateral: A structure away from the midline of the body

Medial: A structure closer to the midline of the body

Metatarsophalangeal Joint (MPJ): The joint that connects the toes to the rest of the foot, i.e., the knuckle

Plantar: The bottom of the foot

Plantarflexion: Movement of a joint in a downward position

Pronation: Outward movement of a joint in multiple planes of position

Proximal: Closest distance from the main mass of the body

Sagittal Plane: Separates the body into left and right halves

Subtalar Joint (STJ): The joint in the back of the foot that allows your foot to move side to side

Supination: Inward movement of a joint in multiple planes of position

Transverse Plane: Separates the body into top and bottom halves

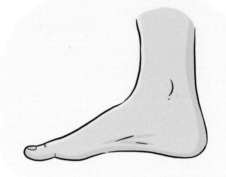

FAQs

Why do my feet hurt?

Good question. The two immediate things that could be contributing to your foot pain are lack of proper support and your body habitus. Poor arch support and obesity can have a direct relationship to why your feet hurt.

Why is proper foot support important?

Without proper arch support, your foot may function in an abnormal position, placing strain on tendons, ligaments, or muscles and causing pain. Having the support of an orthotic allows your foot to function more efficiently and helps decrease the risk of other foot problems.

My parents have bad feet. Should I be worried?

While it is not guaranteed that you will have the same issues as your parents, there is certainly a chance of that happening. Genetics play a key role in people with flat feet or high arches, and both groups tend to have foot problems. Knowing what your family has dealt with in the past regarding their feet and ankles will give you a better history to tell your podiatrist during an examination.

Why is stretching important?

Stretching is a good way to prevent muscle and tendon injuries by warming them up prior to vigorous use. It decreases the risk of muscle strain, muscle/tendon fatigue, and overall injury to the foot and ankle.

How many bones are in the feet?

Each foot has 26 bones in it. The body has a total of 206 bones, so the feet make up one-quarter of all the bones in your body.

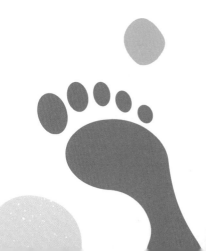

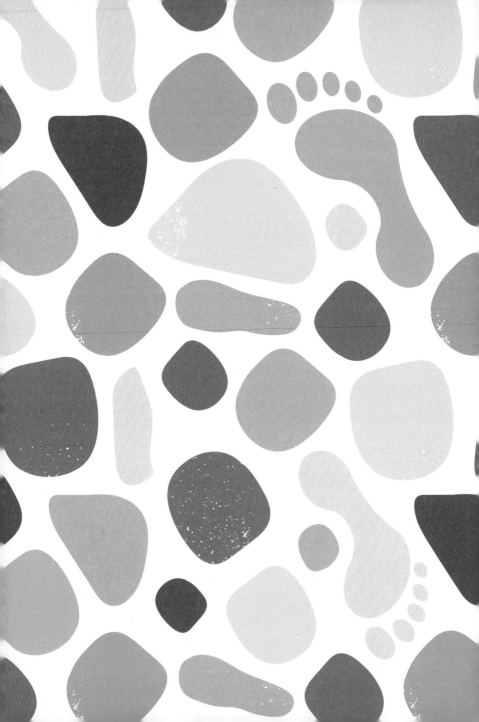

CHAPTER 2

FINDING THE RIGHT SHOE

For some people, finding shoes can be fun, but for people with foot problems it can be extremely frustrating. My patients have gone to the store believing they have found the perfect shoes, only to wear them a few times and discover their new shoes are killing their feet. And the same is true for me. We shouldn't have to buy multiple pairs of shoes before finding the pair that fits right. It can be a time-consuming and costly process. Finding the right shoe shouldn't be stressful, though. In this chapter, I'll discuss some important characteristics that you should look for when selecting a shoe, to make the process of shoe shopping painless.

First and foremost, you never want to rely on the shoe to provide all of the support to your foot. A custom orthotic can provide support, and it can help to lessen the wear and tear on your shoes by keeping the foot in a neutral position, resisting increased forces in higher-pressure areas on the foot. You should always consider adding quality custom orthotics to a good pair of shoes, to increase the support and longevity of the shoes.

Then there is the matter of finding the right size shoes for your feet. A traditional Brannock Device that we used to see in every retail shoe store is not as reliable as it once was, due to the variance in shoe companies' sizing measurements; however, if available, it is a good tool to estimate the size you should be looking for in a quality shoe.

A thumb's width between the end of your longest toe and the tip of the shoe is an easy way to determine a proper fit. If you tend to buy shoes that are too small, they will.most likely rub on your foot, causing pain and blisters. If the shoe is too big, your foot will slide in the shoe, causing you to grip it with your foot and leading to tendinitis and/or hammertoes.

In order to determine the correct shoe for you, first I will break down the anatomy of a shoe by listing each part, which will help you to determine what you need to look for when buying shoes.

THE SOLE. The sole of the shoe is the bottom part that touches the ground. When shopping for a shoe, it is important to look for a stiff sole. A stiffer sole will help prevent excessive rotational forces in the shoe. It also improves the stability of the shoe and prevents muscles from being overworked. Soles that are softer and more flexible allow for excessive use of the foot muscles, to the point where the muscles fatigue, causing pain in the ball or the arch of the foot.

THE INSOLE. The insole is inside the shoe or on top of the sole. This is the inner, lower part that will come into contact with your foot. The insole is probably the least necessary portion of your shoe, as it is designed more for comfort than support. As stated above, when you purchase a shoe, you should not rely on the shoe to provide proper support to the arch of your foot. Usually, the insole of a shoe can be easily removed and replaced with a custom orthotic. Trying to place a custom orthotic on top of an insole, however, can create too much bulkiness in the shoe and make it uncomfortable to wear.

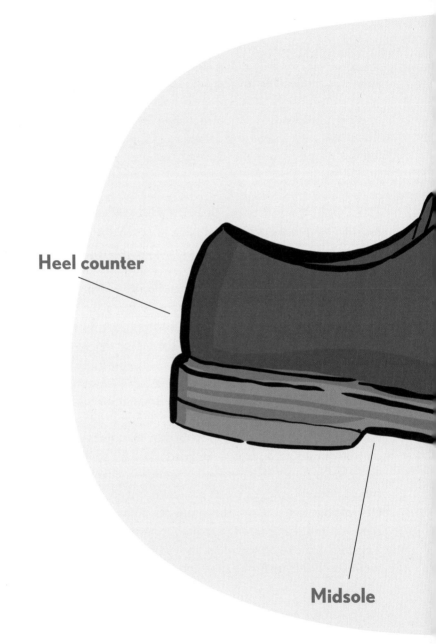

Heel counter

Midsole

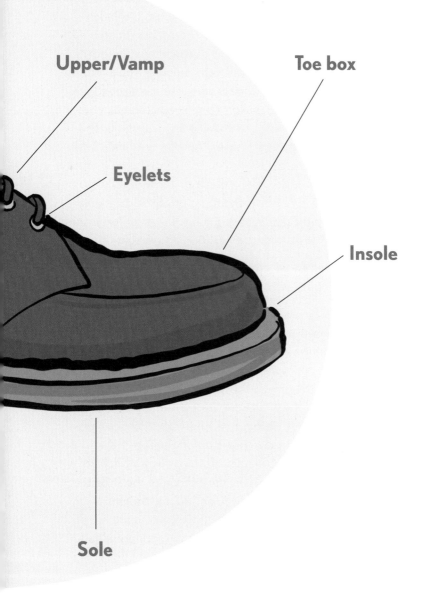

Upper/Vamp

Toe box

Eyelets

Insole

Sole

THE MIDSOLE. This is the bottom part of the shoe at the heel, utilized to incorporate shock absorption. It is below the insole. Many athletic shoes have shock absorption built into them to decrease the amount of strain on your foot when running. Some shoes may have "bubbles" built into the midsole for that purpose, while others may use silicone gel. Having high-quality shock absorption in your shoe can be very helpful when running and training on a regular basis, in order to prevent plantar fasciitis, Achilles tendinitis, and shin splints.

THE UPPER/VAMP. This is the top part of the shoe that usually incorporates the laces and tongue. It is important to ensure that the upper/vamp is not too tight. A tight upper/vamp can irritate the top of your foot, which can cause nerve pain and soreness in the arch, depending on your activities. With that said, your upper/vamp selection should be based on the activities you are partaking in. If you are running and need a lightweight shoe with the ability to let your foot breathe, a mesh-like material is more important for the upper. If you need or want more structure, perhaps in a dress shoe, finding an upper/vamp that is a little more rigid will work better. People with high arches tend to have more pain associated with stiffer uppers and should look for adaptable, flexible vamps that can take pressure off the top of the foot.

THE TOE BOX. The toe box is the portion of the shoe that protects your toes. Having a wide and roomy toe box is important if you have wider feet, bunions, hammertoes, or neuromas. Narrow toe boxes tend to add more pressure and pain to these conditions. The material of the toe box is similar to that of the upper/vamp, and it should be based on your activities. If you are a construction or factory worker, having a firm toe box (steel-toed) for protection is important. On the other hand, if you are playing basketball or exercising, a mesh toe box will provide less protection, but will be lightweight and allow your foot to breathe.

THE EYELETS. This one is rather obvious, but we should touch on it anyway. The eyelets are the portion of the shoe that the laces course through. The most important note in regard to the eyelets is how to lace the shoe if you have a high arch. If you get pain along the top of your foot or have a high arch, skipping eyelets in your shoe can be helpful, depending on where the laces lie, to avoid pressure in certain spots.

THE HEEL COUNTER. The heel counter is the back part of the heel. This is an important part of the shoe to better control your heel and prevent excess motion in the back of the foot. A more rigid heel counter helps control your foot and, to a small degree, your ankle as well. If you pinch the heel counter between your index finger and thumb and it easily collapses, then the heel counter is not firm enough. There should be firm resistance against squeezing the sides of the heel counter in a good-quality shoe.

When selecting a shoe, its appearance, style, and functionality are the qualities we typically assess first, but the support of a shoe should not be overlooked. While I don't expect everyone to wear supportive shoes all the time, it is important to use supportive shoe gear if you are participating in sports or going on long walks or a vacation. To a certain degree, you can get away with a slightly less supportive shoe, if you have proper custom orthotics. However, utilizing the tips provided above will lessen the likelihood of developing foot problems from ill-fitting shoes.

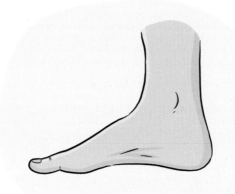

FAQs

Is having a good shoe enough to provide support for my foot?

No, it is not. Having a quality, stable shoe is important; however, adding a custom orthotic is just as imperative.

How do I know if the shoe fits me?

You need a thumb's width between the end of your longest toe and the end of the shoe. If your second toe is the longest, then you should be measuring from that toe.

Why is the sole of the shoe so important?

The sole is important for two major reasons. First, it's the base of stability in the shoe. Having a rigid sole helps to prevent breakdown or excess motion, which prevents foot muscle fatigue. Second, it also provides quality shock absorption when running and hitting the ground during heel strike.

What material shoe should I get?

It depends on what you are using it for. The upper/vamp and toe box are protective and don't do as much for support. If you are using it for work, go with a firmer material like leather to protect your foot better from injury. If you are looking for something to run in, find a shoe that is lightweight and allows your foot to breathe.

Should I run with my new shoes right away?

I wouldn't. Give the shoe time to break in slowly and then progress to running activities. If you followed the points above, you probably have a relatively firm, supportive shoe with little give. If this is the case, it may rub against your foot or heel and cause pain and/or blisters. Break your shoes in slowly and start by walking around your house in them.

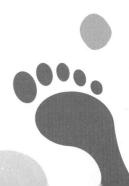

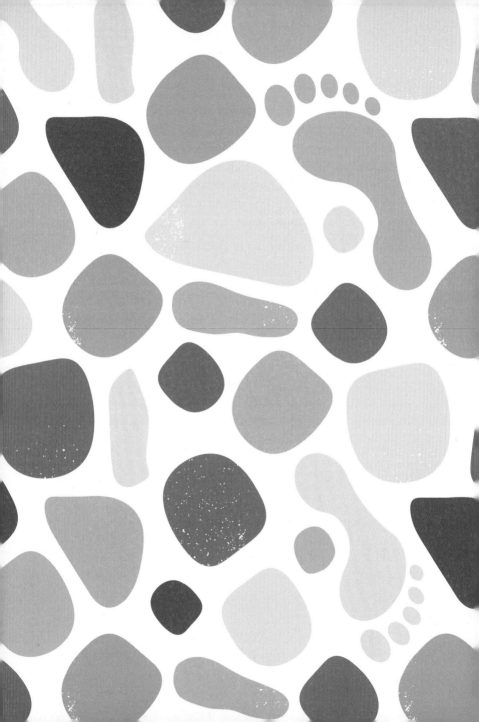

CHAPTER 3

BUNIONS

Normal Anatomy   **Bunion**

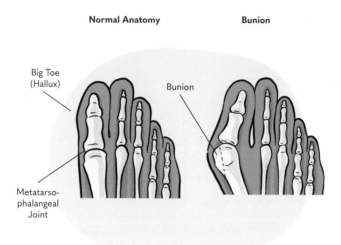

Bunions. Everyone has heard of them, but do you really understand what they are or why you get them? Most commonly, bunions (medically referred to as *hallux abducto valgus*, or HAV) are hereditary in nature; however, there are other conditions that can predispose one to a bunion. Certain arthritic conditions (like rheumatoid arthritis), injuries, or ill-fitting shoes can all lead to a bunion.

Anatomically, a bunion occurs due to an imbalance of muscles and tendons in the leg and foot. Certain muscle groups overpower weaker muscle groups, and the bunion deformity begins to occur. This explains why bunions can worsen over time. This, coupled with improper support, causes the big toe to drift one way and your metatarsal to drift the opposite way of the toe. Ultimately, you notice the big, unattractive bump on the side of your foot. Not all bunions are made alike, and, in fact, not all of them even hurt. Small bunions could be the most painful thing in the world, while large, obvious bunions may not hurt at all. Someone with a bunion may experience burning in their big toe. This is simply due to a small nerve that runs along the bump, which at times can be pinched between your bone and your shoe.

Because bunions are hereditary in nature, if you or a family member has a large bunion, you should be proactive in seeking treatment; this is true for children as well. Early treatment can reduce the likelihood of developing a bunion in the first place, and may prevent the progression of severity.

So, what are your options if you have a bunion? How can it be treated?

Conservative Care for a Bunion

First and foremost, let me make it abundantly clear: the only absolute way to correct a bunion is with surgery. Taping, splinting, and support will **not** correct your bunion. It is a bony problem that requires surgical correction.

When determining options for your bunion, it is always recommended to exhaust all conservative measures before deciding on surgical procedures. The old adage holds true: if it isn't broke, don't fix it. So, if it doesn't hurt, don't do anything about it. Why is that? Well, if you go into surgery with little to no pain, the likelihood of you having less pain, after an invasive surgery, significantly drops. Just because your best friend was back in regular shoes after four weeks and is pain-free, that doesn't mean the same will apply to you.

There are all types of tapes, straps, and splints available on the market to "fix" your bunion. Don't waste your money on these devices unless your goal is to keep your toe temporarily straight, or to give you more padding. As discussed above, you won't magically remove the device one day and discover that your bunion has disappeared. It just won't happen.

Another treatment option, as simple as it may sound, is shoe modification. This may mean avoiding those slides or heels. It could also mean a wider toe box or softer, mesh-like shoes that have some give to them. Probably the most important thing to consider when treating your bunion is support. I'm not talking about the cheap, flimsy inserts you buy at a convenience store or online; I'm talking about a customized orthotic made by your podiatrist. Orthotics are extremely important in the world of podiatry. So what do they do? And how do they help bunions?

The flattening of the arch in your foot leads to the above-mentioned abnormal tendon pull, which can precipitate or worsen a bunion. Having a proper orthotic prevents the dropping of your arch, therefore keeping the tendons in better anatomical alignment to prevent drift. If you have a bunion, an orthotic won't fix it, but it should prevent the bunion from worsening. Remember when I talked about having family members (i.e., kids) checked for early signs of a bunion if there is a family history of bunion deformities? If you can get your child into a customized orthotic early on, you may very well prevent him or her from getting a bunion. If you end up having bunion surgery, orthotics are also a great way to prevent recurrence, because, yes, bunions can return, even after surgery!

Splint devices, shoe modifications, and orthotics. What else is left to help your bunion pain? An anti-inflammatory is a common remedy, whether it be an oral medication, a topical medication, or even a steroid injection. The goal of anti-inflammatories is to decrease the swelling and inflammation around the joint, which lessens your pain.

With the advancement of medicine, other modalities are also becoming popular to help with relieving bunion pain, including laser therapy, shockwave therapy, or stem cell therapy. All of these modalities can be very beneficial, but beware: most of these are not covered by insurance, and they can be costly out of pocket expenses.

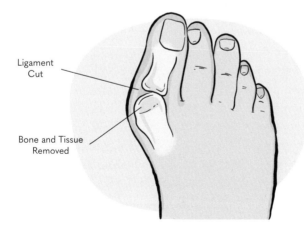

Ligament
Cut

Bone and Tissue
Removed

As previously stated, I would personally not recommend bunion surgery until your bunion pain is affecting your daily life and activities. If you have exhausted all of the above-mentioned conservative options (or at least some of them) and the pain continues to linger, then surgery may be for you. Remember to invest in a good custom pair of orthotics. Even if you have surgery, they will be needed afterward to prevent a recurrence.

All bunions are not made the same, meaning that some bunions are larger than others, and some are more stiff feeling with less ability to move. It can vary from person to person. When determining what type of bunion surgery you need, the surgeon carefully evaluates your foot clinically as well as radiographically (determining what your X-rays look like). Selecting the proper bunion procedure is imperative to reduce the risk of a recurrence.

A larger angle between your first and second metatarsal indicates the need for a more proximal procedure. A more proximal procedure likely means a longer recovery, roughly six to eight weeks. If the angle between your first and second metatarsal is smaller, a distal procedure could be performed, which may only need a four- to six-week recovery. Most recovery times require a couple of weeks of non-weight-bearing; however, this is both surgeon and procedure dependent. A newer bunion procedure, known as minimally invasive bunionectomy (MIS), allows for smaller incisions and immediate weightbearing. A surgical consultation is necessary to discuss which procedure is best for your bunion.

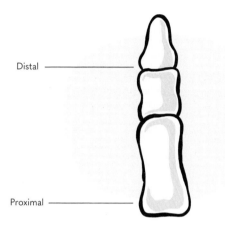

Distal ————————

Proximal ————————

I can't emphasize enough the need to have the proper procedure done for your bunion. If you need a proximal bunion
procedure and you get a distal bunion procedure, I would
say with relative certainty that your bunion will recur, and
most likely will recur quickly. Other than recurrence, what
are possible complications associated with bunion surgery?
Known complications include infection, swelling, pain, and a
nonunion or malunion (meaning your bone doesn't heal back
together or heals in the wrong position). The transfer of pain
to other parts of your foot is also a possibility, because of the
dynamics and the functionality of your foot changing after the
bunion is corrected.

If you decide you are going to undergo surgery, consider
things that will be affected during your recovery. Is it your
right foot? If so, how will you drive? Do you have steps in
your house? If so, how will you maneuver them with a boot

and crutches? Showering will be different, because most surgeons will want you to keep your foot dry until the stitches come out, which is typically around two weeks post-procedure. Reaching those cups on the top shelf in your kitchen may be difficult. So, plan ahead; if you know you will be undergoing surgery, be prepared to have limited functionally for at least a couple of weeks.

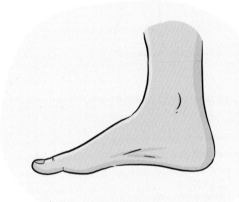

FAQs

Do over-the-counter splints, pads, or straps actually work?

The short answer is no. A bunion is a bony problem, so a soft-tissue splint will have no long-term effect on correcting your bunion. Save your money!

Will my bunion get worse?

It could happen. Unfortunately, your doctor is not a fortune-teller, so it is hard to know for sure, but take a couple of things into consideration. Do either of your parents have bunions, and if so, how bad are they? How old are you, and how bad are your bunions currently? If you are fourteen and you have decent-sized bunions, it is likely that your bunions will get worse. Are you eighty-four with big bunions? If so, what you see is probably what you get.

Do I have to have surgery?

No! Don't let anyone, whether a physician or family member, talk you into surgery. Surgery is permanent. Try the above-mentioned conservative treatments, padding, injections, orthotics, etc., to avoid surgery.

What happens if I don't treat a bunion?

If you do absolutely nothing to your bunion, it will either stay the same or get worse. Throughout my career, I've seen some pretty severe, yet painless, bunions. If that is the case for you, excellent; let it be.

Can bunions come back after surgery?

Yes, over time. A recurrent bunion is actually common. Having the proper procedure done certainly helps decrease the chance of recurrence, as does wearing proper shoes and support following surgery.

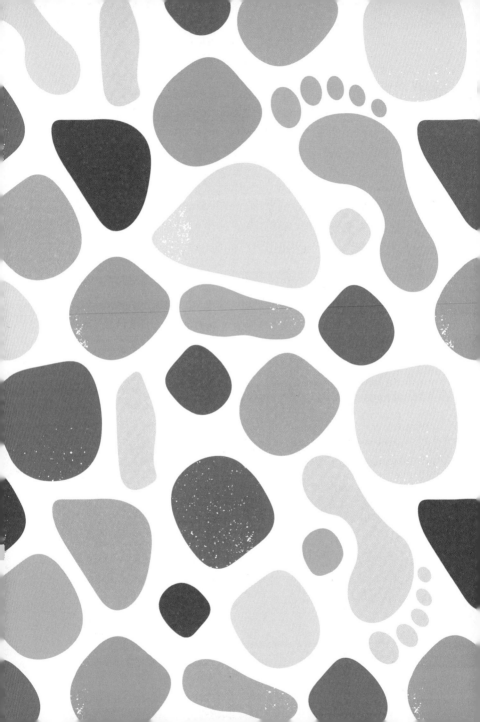

CHAPTER 4

HAMMERTOE

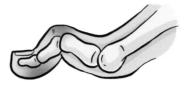

Hammer Toe

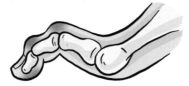

Claw Toe

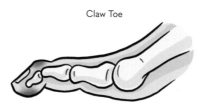

Mallet Toe

Another common foot condition is known as hammertoe. But what is it really? How do you determine if you have one, and how can you get rid of it? If you have a complaint such as "my toe rubs on my shoe and gets irritated," then you probably suffer from a hammertoe. Whether the pain or rubbing starts on the top, side, or tip of the toe, a hammertoe is most likely the source of the problem.

Hammertoes, just like bunions, are usually hereditary in nature; however, arthritic conditions such as rheumatoid arthritis, ill-fitting shoes, or trauma can cause hammertoes as well. "Hammertoe" is more of a generalized term, because there are other subtypes to describe the contracture of toes, including claw toe and mallet toe. What is the difference between a hammertoe, claw toe, and mallet toe? Ultimately, the difference is the joint that is contracted and the position it is contracted in. Hammertoes can be flexible, meaning the toe can be put back in a straight position with manipulation. Flexible hammertoes may not be as painful and can be treated conservatively or with minor surgical procedures. A hammertoe that is stiff and rigid with arthritis to the joints of the toe is typically more painful and requires more invasive surgical treatment measures for the relief of symptoms.

Anatomically, a hammertoe occurs due to an imbalance of muscles and tendons in the leg and foot. Certain muscle groups in the foot overpower weaker muscle groups, and the hammertoe deformity begins to occur. Over time, hammertoes can worsen. A hammertoe can be contracted up and down, side to side, or rotational (see below). Common complaints from people suffering from a hammertoe may be stiffness in the toe, swelling, coloration changes to the skin, irritation or rubbing on a shoe, or possibly a painful corn/callus of the toe. As with bunions, the only way to fix a hammertoe is surgical intervention, since the primary pathology occurs at a joint. Conservative methods such as splints and padding are available to help decrease the progression or help reduce the painful symptoms of a hammertoe; however, it is highly unlikely that these methods will permanently fix a hammertoe deformity.

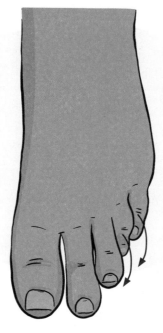

Because of the hereditary nature of hammertoes, early intervention is recommended if you have a family history of hammertoes. Early treatment can reduce the likelihood of developing hammertoes or possibly prevent the progression of severity.

So what are your options if you have a hammertoe? How can it be treated?

Conservative Care for a Hammertoe

First and foremost, let me make it abundantly clear: the only absolute way to correct a hammertoe is with surgery. Taping, splinting, and support will not correct a hammertoe. It is a bony problem that requires surgical correction. When determining options for relieving hammertoe pain, it is always recommended to exhaust all conservative measures before deciding on surgical procedures.

There are abundant tapes, straps, and splints on the market that claim to "fix" a hammertoe. Don't waste your money. If your goal is to keep your toe temporarily straight, to give you more padding, or to take pressure off a painful corn/callus, then these devices will assist in providing temporary relief. As previously discussed, you won't magically remove the device one day to discover that your hammertoe has disappeared. It just won't happen.

Another treatment option, as simple as it may sound, is shoe modification. This could mean using a wider toe box or softer, mesh-like shoes that have some give to them or more space in the front part of the shoe. Probably the most important thing to consider when treating a hammertoe is support. Customized orthotics made by a podiatrist are crucial for providing stability to the foot and appropriate support to the arch, tendons, and muscles in the foot. This support could help to prevent the abnormal pull of the muscles and tendons that cause a hammertoe to develop, by keeping your foot in a neutral position.

What other forms of treatment are available to help your hammertoe pain? An anti-inflammatory is a common remedy, whether it be an oral medication, topical medication, or even a steroid injection. The goal of anti-inflammatories is to decrease the swelling and inflammation around the joint, which relieves pain. Cortisone injections can be cautiously used, in general, for pain relief; however, cortisone may be contraindicated in certain areas of the foot, depending on the biomechanics of your foot and other comorbidities. You should always discuss with your doctor whether a cortisone injection is an indicated form of treatment for your condition.

Surgical Care for a Hammertoe

As stated above, I personally would not recommend hammertoe surgery until hammertoe pain is affecting your daily life and activities. If you have exhausted all of the above-mentioned conservative options (or at least some of them) and the pain continues to linger, then surgery may be appropriate for you. Some patients with darker skin tones experience a discoloration to their hammertoe from the constant friction; however, this is not necessarily a good reason to have surgery. In general, hammertoes are not surgically corrected for cosmetic purposes only because there is a risk, as with any surgery, of complications postoperatively, such as nerve pain and permanent swelling of the toe.

An in-office procedure for a reducible hammertoe consists of a small stab incision, either on the top or bottom of the toe (depending on the contracture). This releases the tendon causing the contracture and allows the podiatrist to manipulate the toe into a corrective position. Afterward, the toe is splinted in the corrected position for approximately one to two weeks. The aftercare consists of weight bearing in a stiff-soled shoe for about one or two weeks. Stitches are not typically needed. There is little to no downtime postoperatively. Usually, this procedure is also more cost efficient for the patient because it is performed in a minor procedure room in an office setting, rather than in a surgery center or hospital. If a hammertoe returns, then you may need to consider the more traditional surgery discussed below.

If your hammertoe is stiff from arthritis or it fails the tendon/capsule release mentioned above, then a more traditional, invasive option awaits. There are several different surgical techniques for a hammertoe correction, which your doctor will discuss to determine the option that is best for you. The two most common procedures for hammertoe corrections are: (1) fusing the affected joint (arthrodesis), and (2) removing the affected joint (arthroplasty).

Usually a podiatrist will use the arthrodesis method for the second, third, and sometimes fourth toe. In this instance, hardware is used to fuse the joint once the cartilage has been removed, whether it be a removable wire that sticks out the tip of your toe or an implanted screw/device. This method calls for approximately four- to six-weeks of recovery in a stiff-soled surgical shoe or a walking boot.

An arthroplasty is usually done on the fourth and fifth toe. When performing an arthroplasty, only part of the joint surface is removed, to allow for the hammertoe to reduce into a straightened position, and no hardware is needed. The recovery is similar to arthrodesis, except there is a shorter time period for healing (approximately two to four weeks).

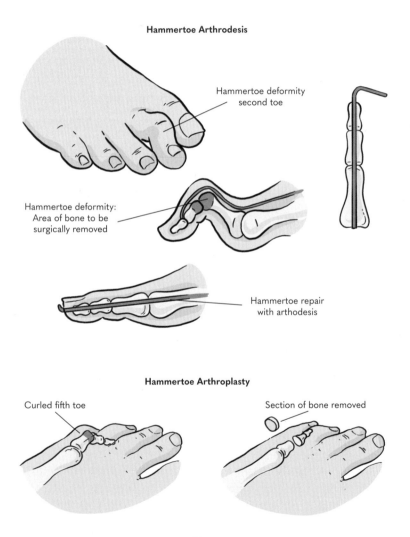

Hammertoe Arthrodesis

Hammertoe deformity
second toe

Hammertoe deformity:
Area of bone to be
surgically removed

Hammertoe repair
with arthodesis

Hammertoe Arthroplasty

Curled fifth toe

Section of bone removed

So why wouldn't you want an arthroplasty on all of the toes, if it involves a shorter recovery and less time immobilized in a surgical shoe? The main reason is that an arthroplasty makes the toe more unstable. Performing a procedure like this on a second or third toe certainly increases the possibility of hammertoe recurrence or a floating toe that does not purchase the ground when walking. Both of these procedures will shorten the toe being treated. Arthroplasties are generally performed on the fourth and fifth toe because they are not primary stabilizers of the forefoot when a patient is pushing off during walking.

Besides recurrence, what are other possible complications associated with hammertoe surgery? Known complications include infection, swelling, pain, a nonunion or malunion (meaning your bone doesn't heal back together or heals in the wrong position), drifting of the toe, and shortening of the toe, to name a few. Transfer pain in other parts of your foot is also a possibility, because the dynamics and functionality of your foot could change postoperatively after the hammertoeis corrected.

If you decide to undergo surgery, consider what will be affected during your recovery. Is it your right foot? If so, how will you drive? Do you have steps in your house? If so, how will you maneuver them with a boot and crutches? Showering can be difficult, because most surgeons will want you to keep your foot dry until the stitches come out, which is typically two weeks post-surgery. Be sure to plan ahead! If you are scheduled for surgery, be prepared for the limitations you will encounter postoperatively for at least a couple of weeks.

FAQs

Do over-the-counter splints, pads, or straps actually work?

The short answer is no. A hammertoe is a bony problem, so a splint will not have a long-term effect on the correction of a hammertoe. Save your money!

What is the difference between a hammertoe, claw toe, and mallet toe?

The difference between these three conditions is based on the affected joints and whether there is extension or flexion at the joint. There are two joints in your toes. Both a hammertoe and claw toe affect multiple joints but differ in flexion and extension, while a mallet toe only affects one joint.

Do I have to have surgery?

No. Don't let anyone, whether a physician or family member, talk you into surgery. Surgery is permanent. Try conservative treatments, padding, injections, orthotics, etc., to avoid surgery.

What happens if I don't treat my hammertoe?

If you do absolutely nothing to your hammertoe, it will either stay the same or get worse.

Can hammertoes come back after surgery?

Yes, there is always a risk for recurrence, due to the complexity of the biomechanics in the foot.

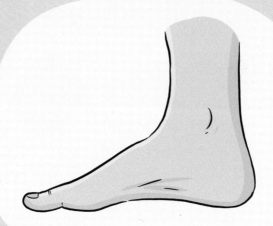

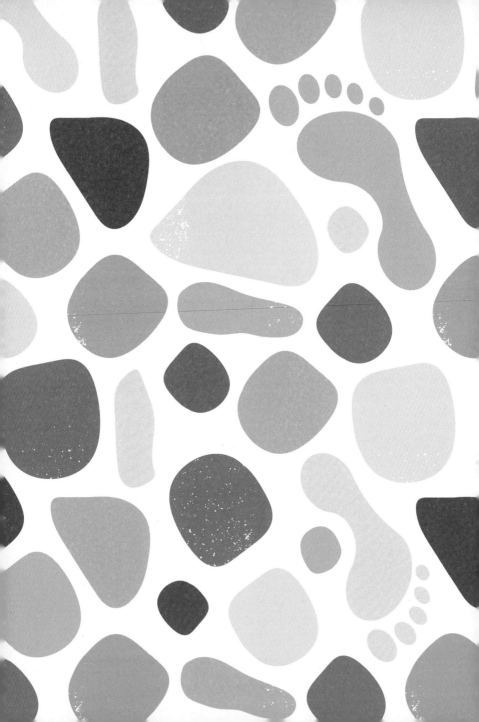

CHAPTER 5

CORNS AND CALLUSES

Everyone has them, and no one can get rid of them. Do you have a corn, or do you have a callus? What's the difference?

Both corns and calluses are excess epithelial tissue that develops on a pressure point on the foot. Typically they are the same color as your skin, but thicker in appearance. Calluses tend to be diffusely thicker spots on the bottom of the foot, unlike a corn, which tends to be smaller, well defined, and with an obvious border. Corns are also most commonly noted on arthritic joints on the toes. They develop because the joint is not moving properly, causing the skin to have an excess amount of pressure in a shoe or against another toe; the constant pressure on the skin will then increase production of epithelial tissue in a single area, producing a corn.

Both corns and calluses develop on a pressure point, whether it is a hammertoe, a bunion, the back of the heel, or across the ball of the foot. Corns and calluses are the body's way of protecting a vulnerable area that is receiving too much pressure. Some can get very large and painful.

Causes of a Painful Corn or Callus

Fissuring: As the skin builds up on the back of your heel or between your toes, the skin can slowly pull away and cause a fissure or crack within it. Fissures typically crack the skin and bleed easily, leading to pain and discomfort. They tend to develop on the back of the heel, especially when you are walking barefoot or using flip-flops/open sandals that do not protect the skin against the shearing forces caused by the ground. It is important to treat fissures, as they can develop easily into open wounds susceptible to infection.

BLISTERING: With repetitive stress and friction to the callus or corn, the skin can separate and a blister can form. The buildup of fluid can lead to more pressure, infection, and pain. Lancing the blister or removing it exposes the nerves in the dermis layer of the skin that can be increasingly sensitive to the touch. Once the base of the blister heals, the callus will likely return if the area has not been appropriately offloaded.

PAINFUL CORE: This can be the case with a corn that develops on your fifth toe specifically. You develop a well-defined corn that appears to have a small dot in the center of it. This is actually a core that can cause pain out of proportion to what you would expect. This type of corn is known as porokeratosis. It can also occur on the ball of the foot, giving you the feeling that you are stepping on something or you have a foreign body in your foot (more on this in Chapter 8). Porokeratosis is the most difficult type of corn to treat, due to its deep-seated core. Even when these difficult corns are surgically removed, they have a high risk of coming back.

So what leads to a corn or callus forming? As discussed above, a corn or callus will only really develop on a pressure point, unless of course you have a more severe skin problem that affects more than just your feet. We will go into more detail on this subject later in the chapter.

The two most common foot problems that can lead to the development of corns and calluses are bunions and hammertoes. Common areas for calluses to appear on someone with a bunion include the side of the big toe joint and under the second toe joint at the ball of the foot. The fifth toe is also a common spot to develop a corn, due to the high pressure of closed-toe shoes and sandals. Hammertoes tend to develop calluses under the ball of the foot, ranging from the second through the fifth toe. The more severe the hammertoe deformity, the worse the callus develops on the ball of the foot or the tip of the toe. Hammertoes can develop corns, either on the top or side of the contracted toe. Do you notice a hard spot between your fourth and fifth toe? If so, you have a corn. Rheumatologic conditions such as osteoarthritis, rheumatoid arthritis, and psoriatic arthritis can also increase your risk of developing corns and calluses, due to the severity of the joint deformity.

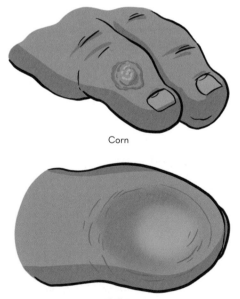

Corn

Callus

Another common condition that can lead to callus formation is fat pad atrophy. All of us have fat along the ball of the foot to give us cushion and protection. Unfortunately, over time, that fat wears down, which leads to the ball of the foot being more prominent. Less tissue padding the area will cause an increase in pressure to the ball of the foot, making it a more susceptible area for callus formation.

Certain dermatologic skin conditions can also cause callus formation. The most common are eczema and psoriasis. Both of these are problems that occur when the top layer of skin produces excess amounts of cells, which replicate layer on top of layer. Typically, these skin areas flake off and bleed, which can also lead to pain. Psoriasis and eczema are autoimmune skin conditions and require care when flare-ups occur.

How do I treat/get rid of my callus or corn?

Full disclaimer: if you have diabetes, it is recommended to see a podiatrist regularly to shave your callus or corn, to prevent cuts, ulcers, or infections.

First and foremost, getting rid of a corn is much easier than getting rid of a callus. I'd like to make one thing abundantly clear: **avoid corn removers**. They don't work. They'll never work. They tend to make things worse. Corn removers contain an acid, usually salicylic acid, which causes the skin to blister and peel. Ultimately this is temporary, because the cause of the corn is still there (e.g., a hammertoe is present). If the source of the pressure is not treated, then the corn will continue to recur.

There are several basic treatment options, which include shaving the corn or callus down with a blade of some sort. Padding and shoe modifications can also provide significant relief from a painful corn or callus. At home, it is recommended to use a pumice stone after showering, when the callus or corn is soft, to help remove some of the excess skin. Be very cautious with the cheese-grater contraptions advertised in magazines or online, as they can be used too aggressively and cause a wound to develop.

Using padding is also helpful in alleviating pressure points. If you have a corn on the top or side of your toe, gel toe sleeves can be used as a buffer from pressure. If you have a corn on the tip of your toe, there are buttress pads to alleviate pressure. If you have a callus on the big toe due to your bunion, there are bunion sleeves to pad the bump. Do you have a callus across the ball of your foot? If so, a metatarsal pad could be used to offload the ball of the foot from pressure. I think you're getting the point. There is a pad for every location and every corn or callus of the foot. Just look online or go see a podiatrist to find the right pad for you. These pads, I reiterate again, won't stop the callus or corn from coming back; rather, they slow the process and make it less painful. Wearing wider shoes or shoes with a softer toe box also helps with pressure points and slows the development of the callus or corn.

Another helpful tool is an orthotic or insert for your shoe. Modifications can be used on an orthotic to help alleviate pressure points on the bottom of your foot. Cutouts and offloading pads can help to reduce pressure, specifically on the ball of your foot.

There are also creams available that help to soften corns and calluses, specifically urea cream. Urea is a thick, strong cream with an enzyme in it that helps to break down the corn or callus, causing it to soften. Again, it won't "cure" the callus or corn, but it may soften the area, allowing pads, orthotics, or pumice stones to work more effectively. Wearing a moisturizing sock at night can also help to soften a thick callus. If you have calluses due to skin conditions like eczema or psoriasis, stronger steroid creams or even prescription medications can be used. These are typically prescribed by a dermatologist.

The final treatment option for corns and calluses is surgery. The purpose of the surgery is to address the deformity causing the corn or callus formation in the first place. If you have a painful corn on your fifth toe due to a hammertoe deformity, whether the callus is on the top or along the side of the toe, surgical correction of the hammertoe significantly reduces the likelihood of a corn or callus recurring. Due to the chance of bone regeneration, there is always the possibility of recurrence of the corn, albeit very unlikely.

Calluses, on the other hand, are much harder to get rid of. If you have a callus on the side of your big toe due to a bunion, then correcting the bunion will usually make the callus disappear. If you have a callus across the ball of your foot due to a hammertoe, correcting the hammertoe and reducing the retrograde force at the knuckle may help reduce callus formation. For diabetics who develop chronic calluses, these are considered pre-ulcerative lesions (i.e., the callus has a high potential to turn into an ulcer). These calluses should be aggressively offloaded with padding, inserts, or surgical offloading to prevent ulcers from developing. Depending on your overall health, your podiatrist will discuss which offloading option is best for you.

A large majority of the population suffers from corns and calluses. Both are very difficult to treat, and many times, surgery is ultimately unavoidable. While conservative options are available, as noted above, surgery is typically warranted to correct the deformity that is causing the callus or corn. Your podiatrist should discuss the conservative and surgical treatment options with you to determine what option is right for you.

FAQs

How do I prevent a callus from forming?

If you don't have a callus or corn already, prevention is the best medicine. Being cognizant of your shoe gear and wearing supportive orthotics will help distribute your weight correctly to prevent a high-pressure point.

Can I get rid of my corn and callus?

Ultimately yes, but this typically involves surgery. Corns are easier to get rid of than calluses, and it is typically because the deformity causing corns tends to be an easier fix, and the overall size of a corn makes it easier to disappear after surgical correction.

Do corn removers work?

No. Don't use them; avoid them. They tend to cause blistering and pain and ultimately don't get rid of the corn or callus. In the hands of a layperson, corn-remover acids can cause severe wounds when applied to the skin of people with compromised immune systems, leading to infections and, in some cases, amputations.

When should I see someone about my corn or callus?

The two main reasons you should consult a podiatrist are (1) if you have pain, or (2) if you are diabetic. If the corn or callus hurts you, and you are unable to walk or perform regular activities due to the pain, seek professional help for alleviation of the pain. If you are diabetic, you shouldn't be treating your corn or callus by yourself. Period. People with diabetes are at a higher risk of calluses or corns developing into open wounds called ulcerations that can be very difficult to heal.

Why do they form in the first place?

The short answer is pressure. Because we walk on our feet, corns and calluses are primed to develop there, just like construction workers may get calluses on their hands. If you were to look at 100 people's feet, 99 of them will probably have a corn or callus of some sort.

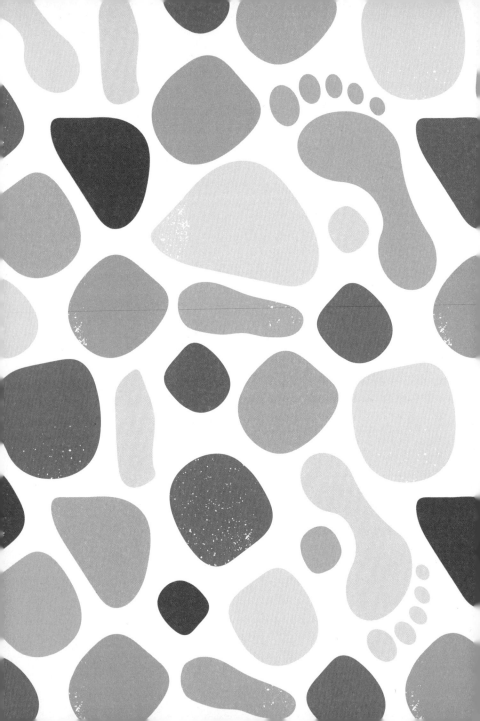

CHAPTER 6

NAIL AND FOOT FUNGUS

One of the most common problems encountered in a podiatry office is, without a doubt, fungus. Whether it involves the toenails or the skin on the bottom of the feet, a fungal infection is one of the most frequent complaints in the field of podiatry. Do your feet itch? Is there a rash or dry skin on the bottom of your feet? How do you get rid of it? Let's go into more detail on how fungus affects the skin versus the toenails and review the different treatment options available for both.

Athlete's Foot

Athlete's foot is the common term used for fungal infection of the skin on your feet. How do you get athlete's foot? You can spread athlete's foot through direct contact, by touching the affected area and then touching another area. It can also be spread through indirect contact, such as coming into contact with the fungus while barefoot at the pool, gym, or karate class. It can also transfer by sharing shoes, such as bowling shoes or gym shoes, with others who may have it. Another group at high risk for contracting athlete's foot are people whose feet sweat profusely and who find themselves in hot, wet conditions on a regular basis.

A little-known fact is that there are actually different types of athlete's foot. The most common type is a red rash that extends around the bottom and along the side of the foot, extending into the arch (referred to as a moccasin distribution). This rash is usually red in color, with multiple small bumps or blisters. Peeling of the skin may accompany the rash. Itching can also be associated with the rash, but it is not always present.

Being in high-traffic areas while barefoot can increase the risk of contracting athlete's foot, whether it is at the gym, in a hotel room, or at the pool. So how do you treat a typical athlete's foot infection? Antifungal topical creams are the treatment of choice, with the addition of a steroid temporarily. The steroid helps to relieve the itching and redness associated with the rash, and the antifungal resolves the infection. It's important to remember that antibiotics (oral or topical) will not resolve athlete's foot. Antibiotics are only used when there is concern that a secondary bacterial infection has developed from untreated athlete's foot. This can occur occasionally in athlete's foot that has been present for long periods of time. It can make the skin appear red and raw around the toes, and it is intensely painful. If left untreated, athlete's foot with a secondary bacterial infection can require hospital admission for intravenous antibiotics.

Another form of athlete's foot leads to maceration or moisture between the toes. One of the more common spots for this to occur is between the fourth and fifth toe on both feet. This is a very common spot for moisture to collect, which causes the skin to break down and become wet. When you look between your toes, you may see white, flaky skin, sometimes with an odor to it. Depending on the severity of the infection, bleeding can also accompany this if the skin starts to break down. This usually forms due to hot, moist environments where the foot is occluded in shoe gear for long periods of time. It can also present in patients with

Athlete's foot is marked
by red, itchy patches
and white flaking skin

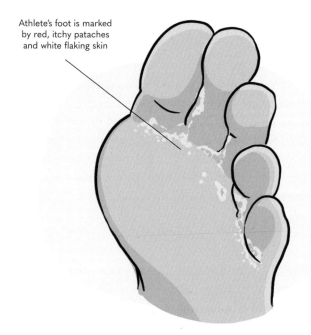

general poor hygiene. Treatment for this includes shoe drying instruments, topical drying agents for the toes, and utilizing cotton-based material (gauze or a wisp of cotton) to keep the toes separated and allow air to circulate between the toes.

For athlete's foot infections that don't resolve with standard topical antifungals and steroid cream, an oral antifungal can be used; however, oral antifungals can have multiple side effects and drug interactions, so a thorough discussion with your doctor is important to ensure it is the right treatment for you. Occasionally, a sample of skin is taken for a biopsy to confirm that the rash is indeed a fungal infection. Although athlete's foot has distinct characteristics, some patients present with a rash that mimics athlete's foot but is another skin condition, such as eczema.

The final type of athlete's foot is called vesicular athlete's foot. It presents as little bumps on the bottom of your feet. The vesicles are usually filled with either a clear fluid or pus. These blisters tend to form, pop, and then dry as a red base that eventually resolves. New blisters then begin to develop, and the cycle starts all over again. In addition to the treatments noted above, warm compresses can be used, and lancing the small blisters as they form.

Fungal Toenails

Finally, the topic that most people have been waiting for... fungal toenails! Fungal toenails may be the most stubborn, frustrating thing to treat in all of podiatry, from the standpoint of the patient and the practitioner. Let's make it very clear: there is no single, surefire way to get rid of fungus on a toenail.

To give you a little insight, it takes approximately nine months for a full-length, normal, healthy nail to form. Because of this, the treatment options aren't quick. They all take time and patience, and when it comes to fungus and unsightly nails, most people lack both. Fungal toenails are typically large, thick, crumbly, discolored, and sometimes painful. The pain is either because the nail is becoming ingrown due to the fungus changing the shape of the toenail, or the pain can

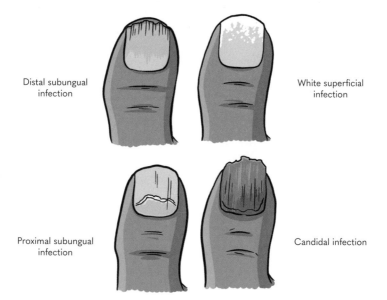

Distal subungual infection

White superficial infection

Proximal subungual infection

Candidal infection

be associated with the thickness of the nail pressing on the skin, causing it to throb. But all thick toenails are not caused by fungus. Also keep in mind that your nail can thicken from trauma or the repetitive microtrauma of a shoe hitting your toenail. Tight-fitting shoes, steel toe boots, and deformities such as bunions and hammertoes can cause unwanted pressure on certain parts of your toes, which can lead to thickening of the nail. Thickness doesn't always equate to fungus.

I usually tell my patients that nails are a window into your health. What does this mean? Well, if you have problems with your lungs, kidneys, liver, etc., your toenails can turn different colors or shapes, or develop lines. Vitamin deficiencies, anemias, and rheumatologic conditions can also make your nails change in appearance. Genetics can even play a role in what a person's nails look like, as people from certain regions of the world are more prone to dark lines within the nails. Why is this important? Because if any one of these conditions is causing your nail to look odd, the fungal treatments won't work. Other treatment recommendations may be necessary, or possibly no treatment at all.

The most basic fungal treatment is the use of topical products. These products, whether prescription, over the counter, or homeopathic, are typically applied to fungal nails daily for up to a year. Yes! You read that right! One year of applying topical products yields moderate success rates (30 to 35 percent).

If you don't have the patience or time for that, what else is available? Another option is an oral antifungal. Overall, the oral medication has about a 50 to 60 percent success rate. This is a pill taken once a day for three months. Following the completion of the oral antifungal, your nail may look the same, because the medication continues to work after you are finished taking it. The medication must penetrate to the cells that make the toenail, which can take months to occur. Once the medication reaches the nail, you may start to notice the base of the nail improving in appearance. During the treatment process with the oral medication, don't be surprised if your current nail falls off; this does happen from time to time. The biggest concern with the oral antifungal medication is how it might interact with other medications you take. And, because the drug is metabolized through the liver, in the setting of elevated liver enzymes, this can cause acute liver failure. Because of this highly concerning side effect, a baseline liver blood panel is drawn before you take the drug and while you are on it, to assure that your liver is functioning properly. Typically, if your liver panel is elevated, simply discontinuing the medication will allow your liver enzyme labs to normalize. If you have a history of liver problems or consume alcohol, it is not recommended to take oral antifungals.

The newest treatment option for fungal toenails is laser treatment. This treatment utilizes a laser to heat and kill the fungus underneath the toenail where it grows. Although patients may feel some heat from the laser, they typically feel minimal discomfort. Several different laser treatment modalities exist, and each has its own settings that vary in temperature and time. While the exact treatment may differ from laser to laser, our office utilizes a laser that typically requires six treatments once a month. And just like other laser treatment therapies, such as hair removal, maintenance sessions may be needed to keep the cosmetic improvement to the nail. Overall, laser treatments for fungal nails result in approximately 70 to 75 percent success.

These three treatment options (topical, oral, and laser) can also be used in conjunction with one another to possibly increase the success rates. Although medical literature is still being collected for definitive evidence, clinical trials have noted that these treatments used together have resulted in more satisfactory outcomes for patients.

Finally, the last option to rid yourself of that ugly, painful fungal toenail is to have it removed. Removing the nail could be done temporarily or permanently. Removing the nail and allowing it to grow back, without treating the fungus, will result in the same nail growing back. Removing the nail permanently will prevent the nail from growing back; hence, no further fungus can reinfect the nail plate. Following the removal of the nail, a chemical is used to cauterize the nail cells, which prevents the nail from growing back. Once healed, it will look like the skin does on top of your foot, or it may develop a small callus overlying the nail bed. Permanently removing the nail improves the chance of being completely rid of the fungal nail 92 to 95 percent of the time. This obviously means there is a minimal chance of regrowth. So, if you want to avoid medications or don't have the time to utilize other treatment options, permanently removing the nail is the best option. The procedure typically heals within 7 to 10 days and is a simple in-office procedure.

So, while treating fungus on your skin or toenails may seem like a daunting task, now you know there are options to potentially clear it up.

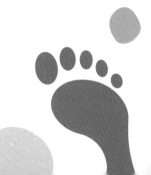

FAQs

How do I get rid of nail fungus?

There are options available, such as topical and oral products or modalities like laser treatments, with mixed results. Removal of the toenail is also an option, but unfortunately none of these options has a 100 percent success rate.

Can fungus come back after I get rid of it?

Unfortunately, yes. Even if you have tried all of the discussed treatment options and finally appear to have cleared the fungus from your nail, toenail fungus can recur once you stop treatments.

Can fungus cause any other problems in my body?

No, it cannot. Nail fungus is specific to the nail plates, so the only other location it could affect is your fingernails. Athlete's foot can develop in other areas of your body. Depending on the anatomical location, it may have a different medical name, but a skin fungal infection is essentially treated the same.

Can fungus spread?

It is unlikely that one fungal-infected toe rubbing on a non-infected toe will cause transfer of the fungus. If you injure a noninfected toe, fungus inoculates the skin beneath the nail because of the weakened or damaged portion of the nail plate being an open, exposed area.

How did I get fungus?

Knowing the exact cause of how a fungus infection started is difficult to determine. Whether it is on the skin or in the nail, you can contract a fungus infection by going barefoot in pools, locker rooms, gyms, or martial arts classes; by sharing shoes; or by injury to the toenail. Fungus thrive in hot, wet environments.

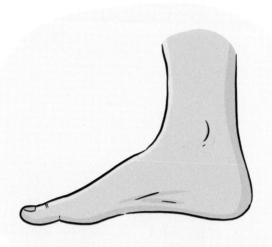

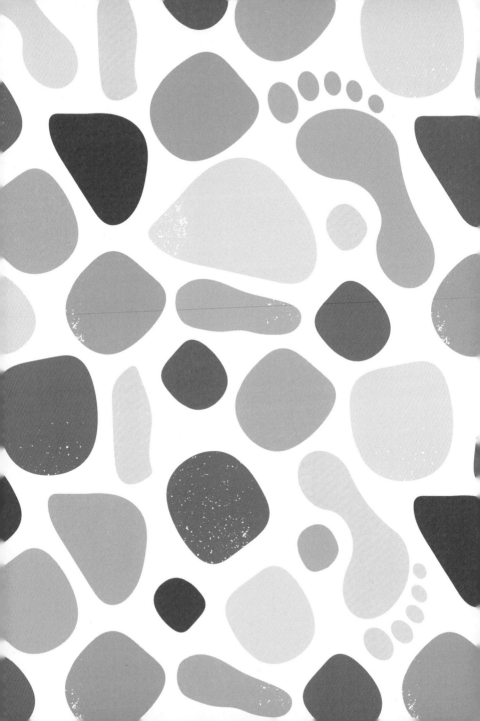

CHAPTER 7

INGROWN TOENAILS

Ingrown toenails may be one of the most painful foot problems. Something so small, yet so painful, can cause an adult to avoid wearing shoes or, even worse, succumb to tears if someone steps on his or her foot.

So, how do you get an ingrown toenail? Probably the most common cause of ingrown toenails is improperly cutting the nail. It is recommended to cut your nails straight across and avoid invading the skin edges at the sides of the nail plate. When you or your pedicurist attempts to cut corners back or dig deep into the nail fold at the skin edge, more times than not a piece of the nail is left behind. Then as the toenail continues to grow, it will grow into the skin, causing pain, redness, and swelling to the skin. Ill-fitting or narrow shoes can also increase the risk of getting an ingrown nail because of the increased pressure on the side of the toe. Other common causes include trauma, fungus, and pedicures. Sometimes genetics play a role in developing ingrown toenails as well. If your nail is curve shaped or you have thicker skin along the side of your toe, you are more likely to develop ingrown nails.

Any toenail is prone to developing an ingrown nail; however, the big toe is the most common location for an ingrown toenail. Conservative treatments like Epsom salt foot soaks and topical antibiotics tend to be temporary fixes. Even having a doctor perform a slant back procedure, where part of the ingrown toenail is removed, is only a temporary fix. These treatments are normally only temporary fixes because the entire side of the nail is typically growing into the skin, not just the corner you can actually see. The side of the nail or the "corner" may be the most painful location, because the sharp spike at the nail is typically missed when trying to fix it at home in your bathroom or at a nail salon. Cutting a V in the center of your nail—an old wives' tale that some swear by, but that has little to no medical evidence that it helps—is of little use either. The nail grows from back to front, not side to side; therefore, the V-shaped cut will not resolve the issue. There are even some newer devices available that claim to help straighten or flatten an ingrown toenail to help get rid of it. Again, this is simply not true and will most likely cause more injury to your nail.

The severity of the ingrown toenail can determine whether an oral antibiotic may be needed. Believe it or not, leaving an ingrown nail untreated can cause an infection, which in rare cases can make you septic (an infection in the bloodstream that can require intravenous antibiotics). So while the condition may seem inconsequential, it's best to turn to a podiatrist to treat an ingrown toenail.

Ingrown toenails can be temporarily or permanently removed. Temporary removals are usually only performed if a specific incident caused the nail and the skin around the nail to become inflamed. An example would be someone developing an ingrown toenail from their cleats during a soccer game. If the ingrown nail has slowly started developing without any specific reason, or has recurred several times, then a permanent removal is the treatment of choice. The key difference between a temporary and permanent ingrown toenail removal is the application of a chemical during a permanent procedure that kills the cells that make the toenail. Therefore, removing an ingrown toenail temporarily will most likely result in recurrence down the road. Permanent removal is the best treatment choice available to decrease the risk of an ingrown toenail coming back; however, as with most medical procedures, there is no 100 percent guarantee that it will never come back. There is roughly a 5 to 8 percent chance of recurrence with a permanent ingrown toenail removal. Some people can be resistant to the chemical used (most commonly phenol or sodium hydroxide) and may need a longer application of the chemical for it to be effective.

Most ingrown nails can be corrected with a procedure called a partial nail avulsion. Usually the ingrown border can be removed while leaving the rest of the nail intact and unharmed. If both sides of your big toe have painful ingrowns, then both sides can be removed and a central portion of the nail plate can be left intact. The in-office procedure starts by numbing the patient's toe. Then, the offending ingrown nail border is freed up from the surrounding tissue and removed, utilizing a special instrument that can get under the nail plate to clip the ingrown out. Once the ingrown is removed, either phenol or sodium hydroxide is applied to the back of the nail fold to kill the nail cells, lessening the likelihood of recurrence.

When would you want the entire nail removed? If you have a large fungal toenail that is becoming ingrown, some people prefer to remove the entire nail versus having a small fungal nail. Another reason would be if you have an ingrown on a smaller nail other than the big toe. Removal of the border on a smaller nail will make the nail on a lesser toe (toes two, three, four, and five) significantly smaller, making it nearly impossible to remove the ingrown without disrupting the rest of the toenail.

Something worth noting: If you have a young child or a special needs patient with an ingrown toenail, try soaking with Epsom salt, apply an antibiotic ointment to the skin, and apply cotton under the corner of the ingrown nail to see if that helps improve the pain and redness associated with an ingrown toenail. While the chances of this permanently fixing a painful ingrown toenail are low, it is still worth attempting prior to any invasive procedures for children or adults with special needs. If all in-office and conservative treatment options have failed, most offices work closely with surgery centers or a hospital that can assist with keeping the patient comfortable with light sedation while performing the procedure. I personally will take my young patients, or those with autism, to a surgery center where a light sedation with gas anesthesia can be used, which helps keep the patient relaxed and pain-free during the entire procedure, alleviating the anxiety associated with surgical procedures in the office. It is a win-win for the patient, the parent/guardian, and the doctor.

Improper cuts   **Proper cut**

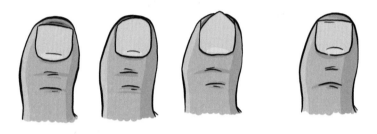

Short   Rounded   V-shaped   Straight

Some patients develop excess tissue on the sides of the ingrown nail, called proud flesh or a granuloma. In this instance, sometimes the skin itself needs to be excised in addition to removal of the nail. Most of the time, there is no need for stitches when the granuloma is excised; however, some providers may apply a couple of stitches if the granuloma is deep or bleeding and cannot be controlled with pressure postprocedure.

What risks can one expect to be associated with ingrown toenail procedures? Common risks include infection, a postoperative delayed healing of the wound, blistering to the skin, a deformed toenail from trauma associated with the procedure, or even recurrence of an ingrown toenail. Although these risks are low, it is still worth discussing any concerns you might have with your doctor. It is common to have some local redness, swelling, blistering and even drainage following the ingrown nail removal, because of the irritation from the chemical used to kill the ingrown portion of the nail. Typically, these postprocedure reactions heal within two weeks, pending no comorbidities or other problems that could slow the healing process. Patients with compromised immune systems, such as people with diabetes, rheumatoid arthritis, or HIV, should talk with their podiatrist to weigh the risks and benefits of having an ingrown toenail removal, with or without chemical cauterization. Those with immunocompromised systems or with poor blood flow can have a delay in postprocedure healing, increasing the risk of infection or a nonhealing wound.

Once the procedure is completed, the aftercare is actually quite simple. Apply an antibiotic ointment to the procedure site and change the bandage daily for two weeks. For the most part, the pain is controllable with Tylenol or ibuprofen. You will want to avoid water areas, such as pools, oceans, or spas during a pedicure, to decrease the risk of infection until the site is fully healed. Activities are not typically limited and are case specific, based on the patient's tolerance level. Ultimately, ingrown nails are very common and very painful. If you have an ingrown toenail, consult a podiatrist for a quick, easy removal and long-term relief.

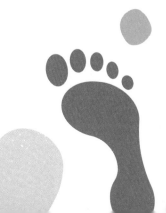

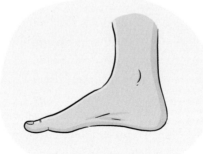

FAQs:

How do you get an ingrown toenail?

There are multiple ways to develop an ingrown toenail. The most common reason an ingrown toenail occurs is improper nail cutting or cutting too aggressively into the skin by the nail. Other reasons are tight-fitting shoes, the way the nail is shaped, trauma to the nail, or fungus that deforms the nail border.

Can ingrown toenails resolve without surgery?

Rarely. Temporary removal of the ingrown toenail can be done by cutting the edge of the ingrown nail out; however, there is a great likelihood of it recurring as the nail grows. Most ingrown toenails require removal by a podiatrist with a procedure that can temporarily or permanentlyremove the ingrown nail.

Are ingrown toenails always infected?

No. The redness and swelling first noted at the site of an ingrown toenail are usually just inflammation from the constant pressure of the nail pushing on the skin. However, ingrown toenails can easily become infected when the ingrown side of the nail pierces the skin, introducing bacteria that can cause infection. If your ingrown toenail becomes severely red and swollen with yellowish or brown drainage, your doctor may require you to take antibiotics to improve the infection, in addition to having the ingrown nail removed.

Can ingrown toenails come back after surgery?

Yes. The percentage is low, at only 3 to 5 percent; however, it is possible. If the nail is fungal or has any type of trauma to it that would affect the growth of the nail, it could increase the risk of recurrence. Also, some people are not as sensitive to the chemical agent used to chemically cauterize the nail cells when an ingrown nail is removed, therefore increasing the risk of it coming back again.

Do children get ingrown toenails?

Yes. Very often, children may not tell you something is wrong with their feet. But you may notice them limping in shoe gear, or maybe they won't let you look at their foot because they're embarrassed or worried that there is an issue. Children are oftentimes afraid to speak up when something is wrong, which is why it is important to ask or watch for general signs of a foot problem.

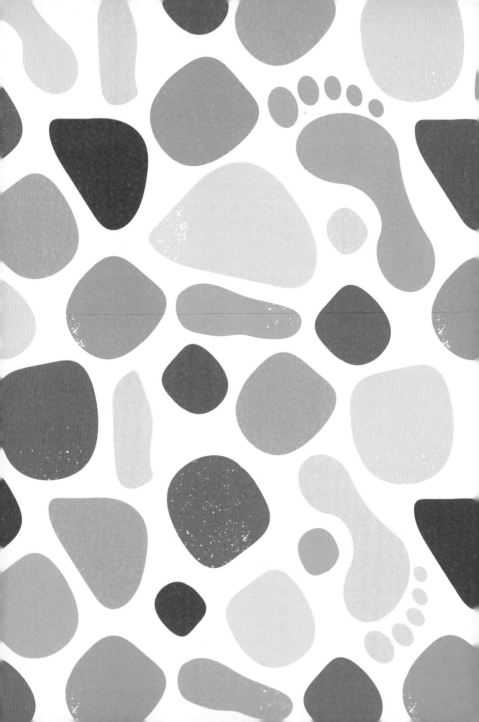

CHAPTER 8

BALL OF FOOT PAIN

A very common complaint I hear from patients in my office is pain across the ball of the foot. The word metatarsalgia is a generalized term used by all podiatrists to describe pain in the ball of the foot. Metatarsalgia doesn't necessarily describe a condition; rather, it's a location of the foot that hurts. Below are a couple of descriptive ways that people use to describe ball of foot pain:

- **I feel like I'm stepping on a marble.**
- **I feel like there is a rock under my foot.**
- **I feel tingling in my toes.**
- **I notice there is a hard area across the ball of my foot.**
- **It feels like there is a sock bunched up in my foot.**
- **It feels like something is popping in my toes.**

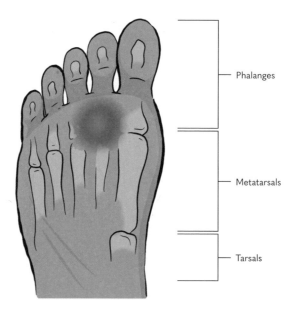

Phalanges

Metatarsals

Tarsals

As we progress through this chapter, I will explain the symptomatic complaints above and talk about how to treat them.

Neuroma

Probably one of the more common causes of ball of foot pain is a neuroma. Despite what the name may suggest, a neuroma is not a tumor. It is inflammation of a nerve that occurs where the metatarsals in the foot and the toes articulate. Specific symptoms associated with neuroma pain are described as "it feels like I'm stepping on a marble" and "I feel a popping in my toes." These symptoms worsen as the inflammation of the nerve intensifies, causing the nerve fibers to enlarge. Once the nerve has become bigger than the space it occupies between the metatarsals, patients will start to notice symptoms slowly manifest and progressively worsen. Common symptoms that help a podiatrist diagnose a neuroma include: pain elicited between the metatarsal heads when examining the foot; pain with compression of the metatarsal heads when squeezing the ball of the foot; a popping or clicking sensation with compression of the metatarsal heads; tingling to the affected toes; and, sometimes, splaying or separation of the toes. While X-rays will not show a neuroma, an MRI or ultrasound may be useful imaging modalities to further obtain the proper diagnosis. However, because soft tissue imaging in the foot can be extremely difficult to perform, even these diagnostic modalities can be flawed. Ultimately, a neuroma is diagnosed clinically by an astute podiatrist, not with imaging.

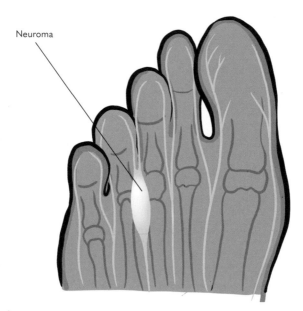

Neuroma

There are four interspaces between the toes, and the most common areas for a neuroma to form are between the second and third toes, as well as between the third and fourth toes. Some of the common causes of neuromas include: tight-fitting shoes and/or high-heel shoes that squeeze the front of the foot; improper support that causes excess pressure to the ball of the foot; and repetitive stress to the ball of the foot with activities like squatting down. Women are much more likely to get neuromas because of the aforementioned causes, but men can suffer from them as well.

So if you have a neuroma, how can you fix it? Just like everything else in podiatry, there are both conservative and surgical options for treatment.

Conservative options are meant to alleviate pressure and decrease inflammation to the nerve itself. Treatment options such as wearing shoes with wider toe boxes, orthotics, and metatarsal pads are all helpful for alleviating pressure on the painful nerve to stop the irritation of the nerve.

If changing shoe gear and using padding don't work, then treatment could progress to injections, of which there are two types. The first is the commonly used cortisone injection, which could require multiple injections, depending on the severity of pain. Cortisone injections use a corticosteroid to decrease inflammation at the neuroma, therefore relieving pain. If the pain persists after three cortisone injections, then we progress to the second option, sclerosis (or alcohol) injections. The alcohol injections are meant to "kill" the thickened nerve fibers from the neuroma and allow regeneration of healthy nerve tissue. Medical literature suggests it may take up to seven injections for complete resolution of these symptoms, so one must be patient during the course of this treatment. If conservative treatment fails, then surgical intervention may be required.

Surgical treatments for a painful neuroma consist of a neurectomy and a decompression of the nerve. A neurectomy is the complete excision of the neuroma; cutting out the thickened area of the nerve leaves a large space between the ends of the nerve, so that nerve regeneration does not occur. A decompression of the nerve is a surgical option that releases a ligament deep in the interspace that helps alleviate excess pressure within the interspace without violating the nerve. The procedures are usually performed with an incision on the top of the foot; however, a neurectomy can also be performed on the bottom (plantar) surface of the foot. Typically, aftercare for either procedure is two to four weeks in a postoperative shoe or walking boot. It can take up to six to eight weeks to feel relief, depending on how much swelling persists postoperatively. The main goal of this procedure is alleviating pain; however, numbness is likely to occur in the affected area. Most patients who suffer from a neuroma gladly accept the postoperative numbness, rather than experiencing the sharp, shooting pain of a neuroma.

The most worrisome complication with a neuroma excision is a stump neuroma. A stump neuroma occurs at the end of the nerve that was cut during the neuroma excision procedure and can cause similar symptoms as the original neuroma, making it seem like the neuroma has returned. While this complication is unlikely, it can cause symptoms just as painful or more painful than the original neuroma, requiring a return to the operating room for revision surgery. Other complications include infection, swelling, hematoma formation, or drifting of the toes.

The final surgical option for neuroma pain is cryosurgery. This is a specialized procedure done only by a small group of physicians in the world. Cryosurgery is an alternative to traditional surgery, and it is done in the office under local anesthetic. It is a minimally invasive procedure where a probe is inserted into the interspace where the neuroma is located; the affected nerve is frozen, stopping the inflammatory process and allowing internal healing and regeneration. No stitches are required. The recovery consists of wearing a walking boot for approximately two weeks. Because this is a regeneration process, patients may not notice results immediately. It may take a couple of months to notice full results, because of the time it takes for regeneration of the nerve. Cryosurgery is not typically covered by insurance. Complications associated with this procedure are minimal. If the procedure doesn't work, then traditional neuroma surgery may need to be discussed with your podiatrist.

Fat Pad Atrophy

Another common cause of ball of foot pain is fat pad atrophy. This problem tends to be more common among the geriatric population. The fat pad on the ball of the foot provides a cushion and protection of the bones and joints, allowing for proper push-off while ambulating. Over time, the fat pad across the ball of the foot can become thin and atrophic due to constant pressure. Simply put, it is part of the aging process. Yes, this is one part of your body where you want fat, but you can't keep it! So how does this cause pain?

The fat in the ball of your foot is an internal cushion, decreasing the stress on the metatarsal heads that are deep below the fat on your foot. As that cushion decreases, the metatarsal heads become more prominent, leading to pain and irritation. Some will complain of tingling in all of their toes, which causes irritation to the nerves. As the fat pad lessens, symptoms such as tingling, burning, or numbness can become more pronounced. The difference between fat pad atrophy and a neuroma is that neuroma pain tends to be more localized, while fat pad atrophy pain is more diffuse. While this is a very common issue, treatment options are limited.

Simple modifications like always wearing shoes and using padding to the ball of the foot are easy ways to bulk up the cushion below the toes. Another newer option is fat fillers. Yes, just like the fillers you can get in your lips or elsewhere on the body, fat fillers are becoming increasingly popular for fat pad atrophy. After a small amount of a local anesthetic is injected, the filler is injected into the ball of the foot, replacing the atrophic fat pad. The downsides to this procedure are the cost and how long it lasts. Unlike a lip filler, a fat pad atrophy filler is on the bottom of your foot, so you are constantly walking on it; therefore, it will wear down much quicker. This will require you to get subsequent injections on a continual basis to help keep the area full and provide an adequate cushion.

Capsulitis, Tendinitis, and Bursitis

I'm lumping these three things together because, honestly, to tell the difference between one or the other is difficult, and they are all treated the same way. The anatomy of the metatarsal phalangeal joint construct is such that all of these structures (tendons, ligaments, and joint capsules) are within millimeters of one another, and the treatments for all three don't significantly change. A positive aspect about all three is that surgery is not typically a treatment option, unless these pathologies are caused by an underlying problem (more on that later).

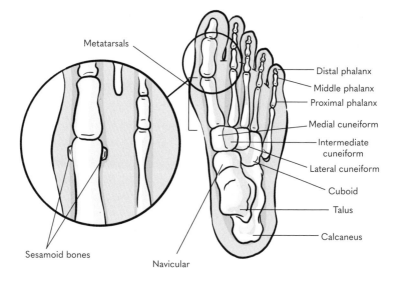

Metatarsals

Distal phalanx

Middle phalanx

Proximal phalanx

Medial cuneiform

Intermediate cuneiform

Lateral cuneiform

Cuboid

Talus

Calcaneus

Sesamoid bones

Navicular

The joint capsule, tendons that cross the joint and the bursa (fluid cushioning of the joint), can cause swelling in the ball of your foot and can lead to that "lump" patients experience. To put it simply, all three of these—the capsule, tendon, or bursa—are inflamed due to excessive pressure or force in the ball of the foot. That inflammation leads to pain or sensations that may feel odd in the ball of your foot.

The tendon runs lengthwise along the top and bottom of your toe and controls whether you pull your toe up or down. The capsule is the shell of the joint that connects the metatarsal to the toe itself. Contained within the capsule is synovial fluid, the fluid that allows your joint to glide freely during movement. The bursa is a fluid-filled sac that is a buffer between the bone and the subcutaneous fat, designed to decrease pressure in a high-pressure area, such as the ball of the foot.

Treatment for these three pathologies is aimed at decreasing pressure and alleviating inflammation. Options such as padding and shoe modifications are sometimes the most simplistic ways of resolving the issue. If pain persists, other options include steroid injections, orthotics, anti-inflammatories, or immobilization in a walking boot for a short period of time. If none of these options work, then surgery may be implemented if there is a secondary deforming force causing the pain. Surgery is typically utilized in the form of a bunionectomy or a hammertoe correction to reduce pain or pressure associated with bursitis, capsulitis, or tendinitis at the ball of the foot.

Calluses (porokeratosis)

Metatarsalgia can also be associated with a callus that has a deep core, called porokeratosis. This type of callus can cause a significant amount of pain and can be quite debilitating for some patients, depending on where the callus is located. Refer to Chapter 5 for more on corns and calluses.

Plantar Plate Tear and Predislocation Syndrome

The plantar plate is a thick ligament that runs across the ball of your foot. The purpose of the ligament is to stabilize the forefoot by keeping all of the toes down and purchasing the ground. Trauma or injury to this ligament could cause toe drifting, leading to predislocation syndrome.

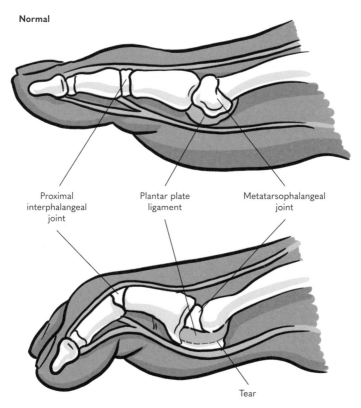

Normal

Proximal interphalangeal joint

Plantar plate ligament

Metatarsophalangeal joint

Tear

Hammertoe

If you sustain an injury to the ball of your foot, you can tear or even rupture your plantar plate, causing the toe to pop up or drift over another toe. Another cause can be a progressive hammertoe where the plantar plate weakens over time, eventually causing the hammertoe to drift over another toe. This will give you the feeling of walking on a ball or marble at the forefoot or cause rubbing of the toe on your shoe. You may notice when you stand barefoot that the affected toe doesn't purchase or touch the ground. An X-ray may show the toe contracted or riding up. An MRI is helpful in confirming if there is a tear or rupture of the plantar plate; however, due to the limitations of an MRI, this is not diagnostic. A clinical exam is the key to appropriate diagnosis of a plantar plate tear.

So how do you treat a plantar plate tear? Unlike many of the other treatment options listed above or in previous chapters, there is minimal success with conservative treatment. Most plantar plate injuries require surgery.

Conservative taping and padding can be used to decrease symptoms; however, these treatments will not fix the injured ligament. Padding is aimed at having more cushion in the ball of the foot, to offload pressure points and prevent rubbing. Taping is used in a figure-eight approach to pull the toe down in a more rectus alignment. By doing so, you should help alleviate some of the retrograde forces causing the pain. Oral anti-inflammatories are also helpful in reducing pain.

I would recommend proceeding with caution with cortisone injections in the metatarsal phalangeal joint, specifically to the second toe. If the area is chronically injured from excessive pressure, then a weakened or injured plantar plate could rupture fully, resulting in a worsening of symptoms rather than an improvement of them. Spending time in a walking boot can also alleviate the pressure and allow the inflammation to calm down to help with the symptoms.

If all else fails, surgical intervention may be required. The goal of the surgery is to straighten the hammertoe and repair the plantar plate ligament. This will allow the toe to come back down to fully purchase the ground. It should also alleviate the "lump" feeling under your foot. The recovery is typically four to six weeks with partial weight bearing in a walking boot.

As you can see, ball of foot pain is much more complex and involved than the term metatarsalgia indicates. So, if you are feeling pain on the ball of your foot and your podiatrist uses the term metatarsalgia, you may want to probe a little deeper into the details of this diagnosis, because more likely than not, you are suffering from one of the above conditions.

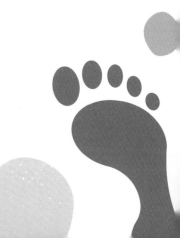

FAQs

What is the lump in my foot?

That lump could be a number of different things, ranging from a neuroma to a cored callus called porokeratosis, to inflammation of the soft tissue structures in the area, such as capsulitis.

Why are my toes numb, tingling, or burning?

As the fat pad lessens in the ball of the foot, the small nerve endings tend to be more exposed to direct pressure, leading to the aforementioned sensations. If it is a diffuse tingling, numbness, or burning, it is more likely a nerve irritation as opposed to a neuroma.

Why are my toes separating?

Toes can separate side to side due to a neuroma formation, which causes the toes to spread apart because of the inflammation and thickening of the nerve. If the toe is elevated and not purchasing the ground, the more likely answer is the weakening or rupture of the plantar plate. Both conditions have vastly different treatment options, so it is imperative to see your podiatrist for a full evaluation.

It feels like there is something in my foot. What is it?

More likely than not, it is a callus with a deep core, called porokeratosis. These little pebble-like calluses can form and cause significant pain, almost as if you stepped on something. Debridement and offloading often help to alleviate the pain.

I don't have any cushion on the ball of my foot. What can I do?

Once the fat pad on the ball of the foot starts to atrophy, there is very little that can be done to get it back. Offloading with padding and using better shoe gear are typically the best options. If these don't work, there are providers that perform fat filler injections; however, these fillers are not long lasting and tend to be costly to patients.

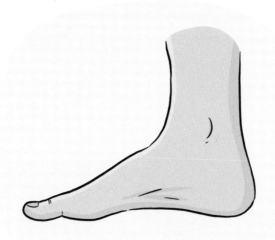

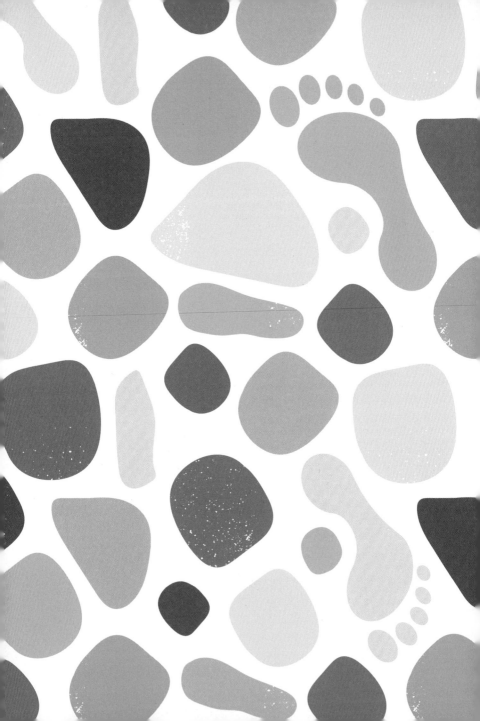

CHAPTER 9

GOUT

Gout is a type of arthritis that is well known but not very well understood. It is commonly misdiagnosed as an infection, which can delay a proper diagnosis and appropriate treatment regimen. So what is gout? How do you get it? How can it be treated?

Gout is caused by an accumulation of uric acid within the body. There are two types of people with gout: (1) those who produce too much uric acid, and (2) those who don't excrete enough of it via urine. Both types lead to increased uric acid in the body, and therefore an increased likelihood of getting a gout flare-up. Middle-aged men are most likely to suffer from a gout attack. While it is rare in younger women, gout is more likely to occur in postmenopausal women. Most of the time gout presents without explanation, such as an injury or an open wound. The pain can be excruciating, and the affected joint is usually red, swollen, and warm to the touch. The most common joints to be affected are the big toe joint and ankle; however, gout can occur in any joint in the body. Uric acid crystallizes within the joint and causes extreme pain. Why does gout commonly affect the feet? Uric acid collects in the joints of the feet because there is less circulation in the feet, and they are naturally cooler in temperature, which allows crystallization to occur more frequently.

So, how do you get gout? While there are certainly hereditary components, the most common cause is diet induced. Foods high in purines, such as red meat, seafood, and alcohol, are more likely to cause a gout flare-up. Although most vegetables are safe to eat, spinach and asparagus have moderate purine levels and should not be eaten abundantly if you have a history of gout. This doesn't necessarily mean that if you eat these foods you will get gout; however, if you are prone to gout, you may want to eat these foods in moderation. If you have gout and you binge on high-purine food or alcohol, expect a flare-up to occur.

Another possible cause for increased uric acid is medication-induced gout. Medications such as low-dose aspirin and diuretics are the more commonly used drugs that can increase the reabsorption of uric acid, increasing the likelihood of a gout attack. Other environmental stressors that increase the body's uric acid levels can be an injury or surgery. If you have gout, always discuss with your surgeon whether you need to take gout medication prior to surgery to prevent a gout attack afterward.

Other than what we briefly discussed before, how do you know if you have gout? Gout is commonly misdiagnosed as an infection. How, you may ask, does someone confuse gout with an infection? When a patient first experiences a gout attack, he or she will typically go to the emergency room or urgent care because the onset is quick and acutely painful. Most facilities will run blood work to check your uric acid levels. Almost every time this is done, your uric acid levels will come back within the correct range of normal limits. This can sometimes lead to a false negative result because the uric acid in your blood has crystallized and consolidated in your joint, therefore causing a false negative blood test. So if you go to the urgent care with a red, swollen, painful big toe joint and are sent home with antibiotics because your uric acid blood work was normal, be aware that gout is not entirely ruled out as the diagnosis. If your pain does not improve within forty-eight hours after starting antibiotic treatment, you should consider following up with a podiatrist or your PCP for treatment of gout.

For the most part, gout is a clinical diagnosis with symptoms such as pain, swelling, and redness in either your big toe joint or ankle, which are the most common "hot spots." Usually, an acute gout attack will be negative on an X-ray as well. Only those who have chronic gout, with many flare-ups over many years, will show definitive arthritic changes to the joint. The definitive way to diagnose gout is by joint aspiration in the office. It can be done during an acute attack; however, it can be painful and is not usually performed unless the diagnosis is difficult to obtain from a clinical exam. Redrawing uric acid blood work after the acute attack has resolved is also a good way to determine what your baseline uric acid levels look like. Patients who have chronically elevated uric acid levels can develop an accumulation of gouty tophi. These are soft tissue masses that, over time, collect adjacent to joints and have the consistency and color of spackle.

So if you have a gout attack, how can you treat it? Typically gout doesn't go away on its own without some sort of medical intervention. Keep in mind that when treating gout, we have to determine if it is acute or chronic in order to optimize treatment.

Acute gout is always treated conservatively. There are multiple oral medications, such as indocin, colchicine, and corticosteroids, that can help alleviate the symptoms.

Sometimes these oral medications may take a couple of days before results are seen. If taken during an acute attack, some other gout medications, like allopurinol, can actually make the attack worse. If you develop an acute gout attack and take a Allopurinol as a preventative medication, you should contact your podiatrist or PCP. They will likely suggest that you stop the medication during this time, and place you on one of the medications listed above for an acute attack.

A quick and effective treatment to resolve gout symptoms is a steroid injection in the affected joint. Yes, the injection will hurt temporarily, but it usually also resolves the pain, redness, and swelling within twenty-four hours after the injection. Avoid applying ice packs to areas affected by acute gout. As stated above, gout attacks colder areas of the body, so ice could worsen your symptoms and actually cause more uric acid to crystallize. A warm compress is actually the preferred modality to assist in reducing the pain.

Chronic gout is treated slightly differently than acute gout. Preventative management is key. Controlling your dietary intake of purines is important to prevent flare-ups. Drinking tart cherry juice is a homeopathic way of trying to prevent gout. There is some medical literature suggesting it helps, but it should not be the primary treatment for gout. Other maintenance medications, such as a Allopurinol and Uloric, are available to take regularly to decrease uric acid levels. However, just because you are on these medications does not mean you can't get an acute gout attack. Patients with severe chronic gout who show evidence of significant arthritis or gouty tophi on an X-ray may need to consider surgical intervention.

As a reminder, surgery could cause an acute gout attack in someone who has chronic gout, especially to your foot. If the

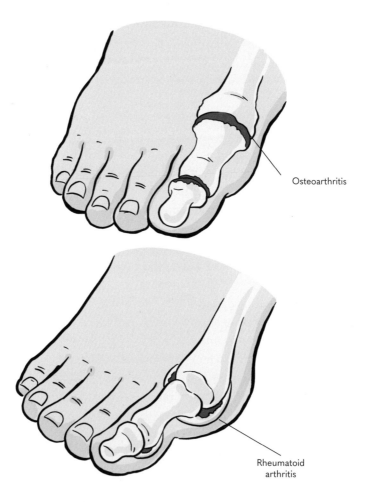

Osteoarthritis

Rheumatoid arthritis

joint affected by gout looks well maintained on an X-ray but you have a large bump on the side of your toe, this could be a gouty tophi collection. Surgical excision of the gouty tophi may be indicated if you experience pain, or if a wound develops from the pressure of the tophi in shoes. Typically, recovery consists of a postoperative shoe or walking boot for about two weeks with partial weight bearing. Surgical excision does not necessarily prevent gouty tophi from accumulating again over time, especially if uric acid levels remain high or untreated.

If you have severe arthritis to your big toe joint, secondary to gout, then there are two surgical options commonly available: fusing the big toe joint (arthrodesis) or a big toe joint replacement (arthroplasty). The fusion removes the joint and motion to the big toe, but it also prevents future flare-ups in that area, because the joint is no longer present. No joint, no flare-up. This is reserved usually for active, younger patients, because it is a long-term fix and can withstand the impact of higher levels of activity. The recovery is approximately six to eight weeks in a boot, partial to non-weight-bearing.

The alternative to a fusion is a total joint replacement with an implant. Implants are usually utilized for older, less active patients, because they can eventually wear out. Although you can retain some range of motion to the toe, it may not be the same amount as a normal toe joint. If you are younger and are considering an implant, expect the need for a secondary surgery in the future to replace the worn-down implant. Depending on the integrity of the joint, another implant can be placed, or a fusion may be indicated at that time. Implants tend to have a quicker recovery of about two weeks of weight bearing in a boot. Gout flare-ups in a joint with an implant are rare but not impossible.

So, while gout can be an extremely painful problem, there are good treatment options available. Be proactive in treating gout early to prevent the chronic phases of the disease process from progressing to an advanced state that is more difficult to treat.

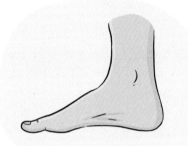

FAQs

What does my foot look like when I have gout?

A typical presentation of gout occurs in the big toe joint in the middle of the night. Acute gout is associated with severe pain, and the affected joint will be red, swollen, and warm to the touch. While it can occur anywhere in the body or foot, the big toe joint and ankle are the most common areas.

What causes gout?

Foods with high purine levels—red meats, organ meats, seafood, alcohol—can cause a gout flare-up by increasing uric acid levels in your body.

Do men or women get gout?

Middle-aged men are far more commonly diagnosed with acute gout; however, postmenopausal women are also susceptible to developing acute gout.

I tried icing my foot to alleviate the pain, but it didn't work. Why?

Gout likes to attack colder areas of the body because the uric acid crystallizes more easily in cooler temperatures. Applying ice can make symptoms worse because it encourages more crystallization of the uric acid. Use a warm compress instead to prevent further crystallization.

I had a flare-up. How bad will my arthritis be?

It depends. If you develop flare-ups occasionally, or less than three in a year, then most likely your arthritis will not progress to more severe symptoms. However, if you have chronic gout with acute flare-ups three to six times a year, then it is likely the joint will become more affected by arthritis.

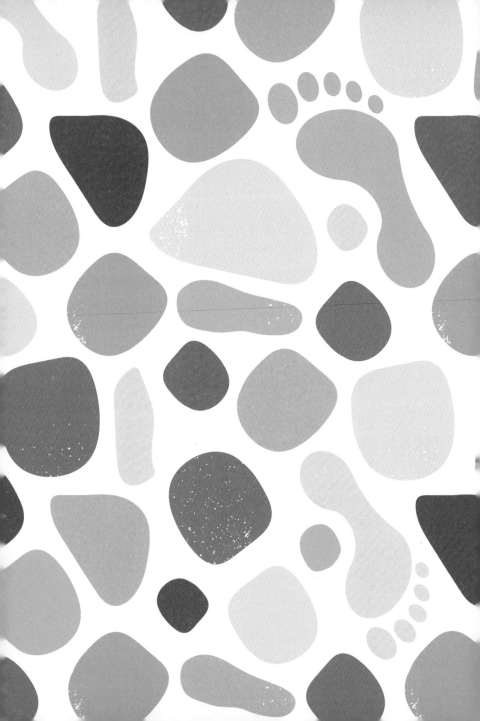

CHAPTER 10

WARTS

A wart, also known as a verruca, is a well-known dermatologic problem that can occur anywhere on the body. The difference between a wart on your hand versus one on your foot is the viral strand. Verruca plantaris is the medical name for what is commonly called a plantar wart. That is it. Just like with any other virus, it is difficult to treat plantar warts, and there is always the likelihood for possible recurrence.

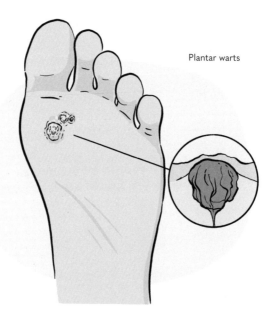

Plantar warts

The word "plantar" is the medical term for the bottom of the foot; hence, a plantar wart is found on the bottom of the foot. Very rarely, warts can be found on top of the foot. How do you get plantar warts? Walking around barefoot in high-traffic areas like gyms, locker rooms, pools, or bathroom facilities allows your feet to come into contact with the virus. It can also be transferred through direct contact. For example, if a family member has a wart, it can be transferred by using the same facilities, or by your family member touching the wart with his or her hand and then touching you. Once you have a wart, it can certainly spread from the initial lesion. Plantar warts usually present as a single, identifiable lesion, though you can develop multiple lesions on one or both feet. A mosaic wart, however, is a large, multinucleated wart that is ill defined and very difficult to treat.

Pain on the bottom of the foot, misdiagnosed as a callus or corn, is usually what drives a patient to seek treatment from a podiatrist. Warts will hurt with compression or with squeezing both sides of the lesion, compared to the aforementioned callus. The best way to truly tell the difference between a wart and a callus is by looking at the base of the lesion after the thicker skin is removed. The skin lines on the foot will go around a wart because it is a foreign virus invading the skin bed, whereas a simple callus will have skin lines going straight through the lesion. Another telltale sign is pinpoint bleeding to the wart after the top layer of skin has been removed. The removal of the thicker tissue that your body produces in reaction to the virus exposes the small vascular network the virus has created, causing pinpoint bleeding to occur. You may see little black dots as well, which are spots of dried blood from the vasculature of the virus. So don't worry if you are trying to treat a wart and it bleeds; this is very common and usually suggests you are at the base of the virus. Warts are contained within the skin only and do not penetrate any deeper into the foot or body.

There are multiple treatment options to resolve a stubborn wart. Some are more conservative than others. The most basic form of treatment is salicylic acid and duct tape. Yes, you read that correctly: duct tape. The same type of tape that can fix anything in your house may also be able to treat your wart. Why duct tape? Literature suggests that duct tape has strong adhesive properties that can prevent oxygen from getting to the wart while it is being treated. Another advantage to using duct tape is that it will peel some of the dead tissue away with each removal and reapplication, meaning that the thick tissue built up on the wart will be pulled away continually, leaving the base of the wart occluded with the tape. When treating with salicylic acid, only apply a small amount to the wart itself. This is important. If you apply too much, the chemical can spread to normal, healthy skin, causing it to break down as well. Avoid presoaked pads, as they usually go beyond the surface area of the wart, leaving you with irritated, blistered skin. How long will it take it to go away? It truly varies per individual. I've treated some warts that go away in two weeks; however, I've also treated other patients for months before improvement was noted.

Some practices offer to freeze the wart with liquid nitrogen, which kills the wart by causing it to blister and fall off. It is difficult to utilize this form of treatment with plantar warts, as some warts are deeper in the skin, and the liquid nitrogen cannot penetrate the entire depth of the wart. A product called Cantharidin is commonly used for plantar warts. Cantharidin is actually a liquid extracted from the Cantharidin beetle. Yes, beetle juice. Cantharidin is applied to the wart with a small cotton-tip applicator. An adhesive bandage is then used to cover the wart daily, until a follow-up with your podiatrist in two weeks. Around the third to fifth day, the application site will blister, causing moderate pain that slowly subsides. During the follow-up, your podiatrist will shave the blister to the point where it peels off like a sticker. For most patients, after two weeks the wart will be gone, and the skin must regenerate where the previous wart was noted. This can take an additional two to four weeks, depending on the patient and the size of the original wart.

The last form of treatment is excision of the wart. Cutting out the wart is definitely the most aggressive option, but it is the most effective treatment method. This can be done in the office or in a surgery center if sedation is required. A local anesthetic is used to ensure that the patient doesn't feel anything at the site of the wart. Once the patient is numb, a small blade is used to excise the wart. Stitches are not normally needed following an excision because the wart is housed within the skin layer only.

What are the typical characteristics your podiatrist is looking for, to know the wart has been removed in total? There are actually two ways of knowing. One is dependent on the bleeding. If wart tissue is still present, pinpoint bleeding will continue to occur. If the wart tissue has been fully excised, no further pinpoint bleeding will be noted. The second is the consistency of the tissue being removed. Oddly enough, when cutting out the wart, it looks and feels like celery. Evaluating the skin and surrounding tissue to make sure only normal, healthy skin tissue is present is an important aspect of surgically removing a wart. Following the excision, silver nitrate is applied to cauterize the bleeding, and a dressing is applied to the foot. The patient will change the dressing daily for the next two weeks, with a follow-up visit afterward to ensure that good healing is noted on the residual skin.

Oral medications have also been helpful as off-label uses for the treatment of warts. We will start some older patients on a month's supply of cimetidine. Cimetidine is an acid reducer used for heartburn. Oddly enough, there are studies that prove cimetidine is successful in helping the body rid itself of the virus that causes a wart. This isn't normally recommended for younger patients, as it is not a first-line treatment for a young, healthy individual. When cimetidine is prescribed, we usually instruct the patient to take it three times a day for one month, and then have a follow-up visit for further evaluation.

There are other topical treatments, such as 5-fluorouracil and retinoid products, that have been utilized off-label for wart treatment; however, further study is still needed to evaluate the efficacy of these products.

Yes, warts are very stubborn and tough to treat. Patients and providers can both become equally frustrated when trying to treat warts, since everyone's treatments and outcomes vary. But options exist; you just have to be patient and consistent with the treatments.

FAQs

Are warts contagious?

Yes, they are. Warts are a virus that can spread through direct and indirect transmission.

Can warts spread to other parts of my body?

Yes, they can. Be sure not to touch warts with your fingers and rub other spots on your body. Good hand hygiene is essential when treating warts with topical applications.

Will warts clear up on their own?

Occasionally warts can spontaneously resolve; however, it can take months to even years for them to clear up on their own. Seeking treatment is usually required.

How do I know it is a wart?

After shaving the excess tissue down, there are some characteristics that distinguish a wart from a callus. Pinpoint bleeding and divergent skin lines are the most common identifiable features of a wart.

How quickly will warts go away?

Unfortunately, there is no way to know how long treatments will take to resolve warts because they are a virus.

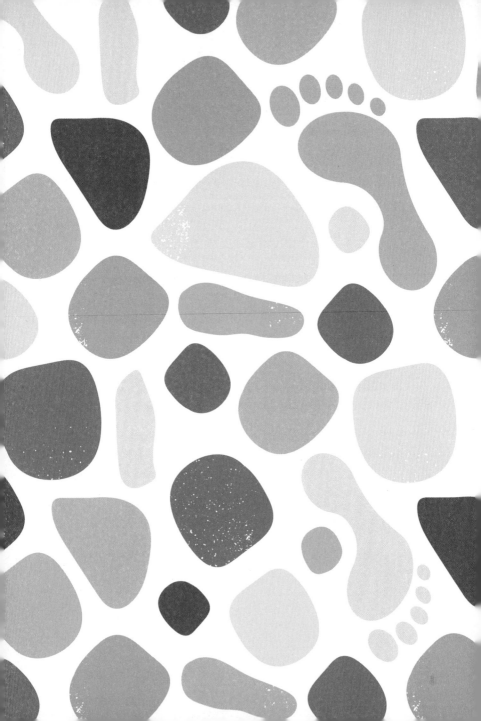

CHAPTER 11

LUMPS, BUMPS, AND MASSES

Lumps, bumps, and masses come in all shapes and sizes. They could be virtually anything from a common, small, benign cyst to a rare, malignant cancer. I'll outline the most common lumps, bumps, and soft tissue masses that can occur on your feet and the treatments associated with them. Thankfully, the majority of the time, these lumps and bumps on your feet are benign issues, meaning they are not cancerous. However, that does not mean cancer does not occur in the foot. Soft tissue cancers, also called sarcomas, and bone cancers have been documented in the foot; however, malignant cancers are rare and are not typically at the top of the differential diagnoses upon initial examination of a soft tissue mass in the foot. An overview of skin cancers can be found in Chapter 20. Refer to this chapter for more details.

To appropriately diagnose a soft tissue mass, regardless of location, it is necessary to utilize a combination of clinical examination and diagnostic imaging. Sometimes a biopsy is warranted, where a small piece of the soft tissue mass is removed and sent for microscopic evaluation by a pathologist. Clinical examination can be very telling as to whether a soft tissue mass is malignant or benign. If the mass is well defined, soft, and mobile (meaning it moves freely on the skin surface), then these features suggest a benign mass. However, if the mass appears to be hard, ill defined, fixed to the skin, and is painful to the touch, these characteristics could be that of a malignant mass, and further investigation should be performed. Imaging such as X-rays, CT scans, and MRIs can be useful as well for finding the right diagnosis. If imaging reveals bony destruction or calcifications near the location of a soft tissue mass, then this is highly suspicious for a malignant tumor. If there are no locally invasive features to the mass on imaging, and it appears well defined, then the mass is most likely benign. Ultimately a biopsy is the gold standard for an accurate diagnosis. Depending on the size of the mass, this can typically be performed in the office under local anesthesia.

Lipomas

A lipoma is the first lump to address because it is the most common soft tissue mass found on the foot. A lipoma, in short, is a benign soft tissue collection of fat. Lipomas can come in all sizes, depending on the size of the patient and the location where it's growing. The most common location for lipomas is the outside of the foot and ankle. They are more commonly noted in postmenopausal women. When examining a lipoma, it tends to be soft in nature and well defined. A lipoma is typically not a painful lump, unless it is pushing on an adjacent structure such as a nerve or tendon. If this is the case, you may experience burning or tingling around the mass itself that can radiate toward the toes. Most of the time, lipomas are more of a cosmetic concern to the patient, rather than a condition associated with pain or discomfort.

Intervention is usually only required for painful lipomas. If the lipoma is not painful, it is best advised to monitor the lipoma and not surgically intervene for cosmetic purposes only. If the mass is painful, then surgical intervention may be warranted. There are no effective conservative treatments for lipomas on a lower extremity. Surgical excision is a relatively easy procedure. The larger the mass, the more difficult the excision may be, due to the increased vascularity associated with larger lipomas. The mass is usually sent for pathology upon removal, to ensure that it is nothing more than a fatty mass. The aftercare is typically non-weight-bearing to partial weight bearing in a walking boot for approximately two weeks, until the sutures come out. A walking boot is important if the lipoma is excised over the ankle joint because the boot prevents constant motion at the incision site, therefore decreasing the risk of the incision opening up after surgery.

Complications for a lipoma excision are relatively low, with the most common complications being those of any surgery: infection, delayed wound healing, or recurrence. If a nerve is entrapped within the tissue of the lipoma, then localized numbness or tingling/burning are also possible postoperative complications that could be temporary or permanent, pending the regeneration of the nerve once the lipoma is excised.

Cysts

Cysts are the next common mass to encounter in the foot or ankle. There are three types of cysts usually seen in the foot and ankle: an inclusion cyst, a mucoid cyst, and a ganglion cyst.

An inclusion cyst usually develops on the bottom of the foot and feels like a small marble under the skin. It most commonly develops from some type of localized trauma, like stepping on something.

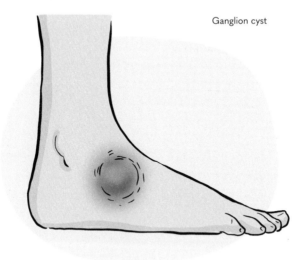

Ganglion cyst

A mucoid cyst develops due to a disruption of the synovial fluid within the joint, and it pops up on the skin.

A ganglion cyst is the largest of the group, and it develops from the joint but also from a disruption from the tendon sheath. Let's delve into each one a little more in depth.

Inclusion cysts are small, firm, pearl-looking cysts that develop on the bottom of the feet. Most people complain of a small mass on the bottom of the foot. When palpating it, the marble-sized mass feels like it rolls around under your finger. Pain is usually obvious because of it being on the bottom of your foot. The development of these cysts may develop following a trauma, e.g., stepping on a kid's pointy toy with relative force. The only way to treat them conservatively is by applying offloading padding around the mass to redistribute the weight and avoid direct pressure. Surgical excision is something that can be done in-office with a small amount of local anesthesia and one to two stitches. Inclusion cysts have a low recurrence rate, and complications as a whole are pretty rare.

Mucoid cysts are usually the smallest of the three, and always develop on the toes. There are two small joints in each toe, and the mucoid cyst normally develops on the closest one to the nail plate. It looks like a bubble on the tip of the toe. It can be painful when rubbing on shoes, or it can just be strictly unsightly and cosmetically unappealing. Most patients admit to popping it with a pin, or it can pop on its own from rubbing on a shoe. The contents of the mucoid cyst are similar to a ganglion cyst, in that they are very gelatinous in nature. The stalk of the mucoid cyst extends down to the joint it sits above. Treatment for a mucoid cyst varies. Lancing the cyst in-office and applying antibiotic ointment is a possibility; however, it will return in a short period of time. In-office surgical excision is another option, and it is done under local anesthesia. The main problem with this is that getting the stalk of the cyst out can be difficult, meaning recurrence is a high possibility. A more aggressive surgery involves removing a portion of the underlying bone, therefore destroying the joint to ensure that the cyst will not come back. The downtime for these procedures is relatively nonexistent, and recurrence is always a possibility.

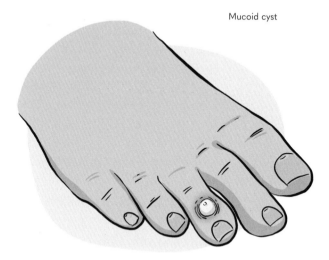

Mucoid cyst

Ganglion cysts are the final type of cyst typically encountered in the foot and ankle. These are usually the largest and most apparent of all the cysts. Like mucoid cysts, they typically have a stalk that extends down to the joint, but they can also develop due to a disruption in the tendon sheath. The most common spot to see a ganglion cyst is the top of the foot or ankle. It feels like a large water balloon when you push on it. The contents of the cyst are gelatinous in nature. Unlike the cysts discussed above, there are conservative and surgical options for a ganglion cyst. Conservative treatment is aimed at decreasing the size of the cyst. In-office cyst aspiration can be performed. Basically, a needle is placed within the cyst and the fluid is extracted via a syringe. Following the aspiration, a compressive dressing is applied to keep the cyst flat for a more extended period of time. Sometimes a steroid injection will be applied in hopes of causing the shell of the cyst to break down and prevent recurrence. Even with this, however, just by aspirating the cyst, it will return. For some patients, coming in every once in a while to have the cyst drained is preferable to having it surgically removed. Surgical excision, which removes the cyst and all of its content, is the final option. The problem with this is that ganglion cysts tend to be much larger than they appear. They usually have many stalks and go in multiple directions. Because of this, recurrence is highly likely. Downtime is approximately two weeks in a walking boot.

Overall, treatments of cysts are relatively straightforward and easy to have done, with very little downtime. Just like any other surgery, complications are always a possibility, which is why it should be reserved until the pain or pressure is not tolerable.

Plantar Fibroma

Last are plantar fibromas, which may be the most stubborn of the aforementioned masses. Fibromas are a collection of fibrous tissue within the plantar fascia on the bottom of your foot, but they can occur in the palm of the hand as well. They can present as small and not painful to large enough that it is difficult to walk. They typically form in the arch of the foot, and can be singular or multiple in number. They are usually firm to the touch and can cause occasional pain. Other than the fact that it is a convex mass on the bottom of your foot, plantar fibromas can sometimes put pressure or wrap around a local nerve, which can lead to pain. Sometimes referred to as Ledderhose disease, there are genetic implications. Another cause of plantar fibromas is repetitive trauma or stress to the arch of your foot. It is common for podiatrists to see this in roofers because of how they place their feet on the ladder rungs that they are constantly going up and down.

Diagnosing a plantar fibroma is relatively easy because of the consistency of the location and the way the plantar fibroma feels. X-rays are usually negative, and sometimes an MRI is used to give you a better idea of the exact size of the mass itself. Treatment options are not very expansive.

The simplest way to treat a plantar fibroma is doing nothing beyond simply monitoring it. If it doesn't hurt, just like everything else, don't fix it. If it is small and not irritating, then don't worry about it.

The next option to treat a fibroma is offloading. A customized orthotic can be made that has a cutout in it to take the pressure off of the mass, which alleviates the pain. Verapamil cream is a topical product with demonstrated efficacy in shrinking the size of plantar fibroma masses. The main issue is that it takes a long time, so don't expect a quick response with the topical cream.

The next course of treatment involves injections, specifically using cortisone. Injecting a cortisone within the plantar fibroma can decrease the size of the mass. This may take multiple injections over time. While they don't feel great, cortisone injections for plantar fibromas do tend to be very successful. There are also Vitrase injections. Vitrase is an enzyme that allows for better absorption of the steroid that is included in the injection. There are some studies that promote the use of Vitrase and its success in shrinking the size of these fibromas.

Surgical excision for plantar fibromas is not recommended, unless you really have no other choice. The main reason for this is because plantar fibromas have a high recurrence rate and typically return larger and more painful than when they initially presented. I would do everything in my power to avoid a surgery like this. The recovery is typically three weeks in a walking boot.

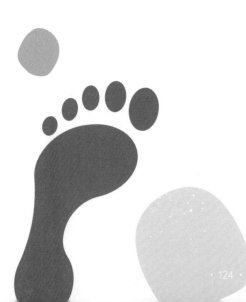

FAQs

What is the bump on my foot?

While there are many types of bumps on the foot, both benign and malignant, most bumps are benign. There is a laundry list of possibilities as to what the bump could be, but the most likely scenario is a lipoma, cyst, or plantar fibroma.

How can I get rid of my fibroma?

There is no guaranteed way to get rid of a painful fibroma. However, options such as topical creams and injections are helpful in reducing the size and the pain of the mass.

How do you get a cyst?

A cyst is formed in one of two ways. One would be from injury or irritation to the joint capsule. A stalk forms and develops a cyst that you see exposed on the skin. The other cause is from a disruption to the tendon sheath, which allows fluid to leak out and develop a cyst.

What is this mass on the front of my ankle?

Most likely it is a lipoma, a benign mass. It is extremely common on the front of the ankle, specifically in heavier patients.

Should I have my fibroma cut out?

No, I would highly recommend against that. Plantar fibromas have a high recurrence rate and typically come back larger and more painful than before the surgery.

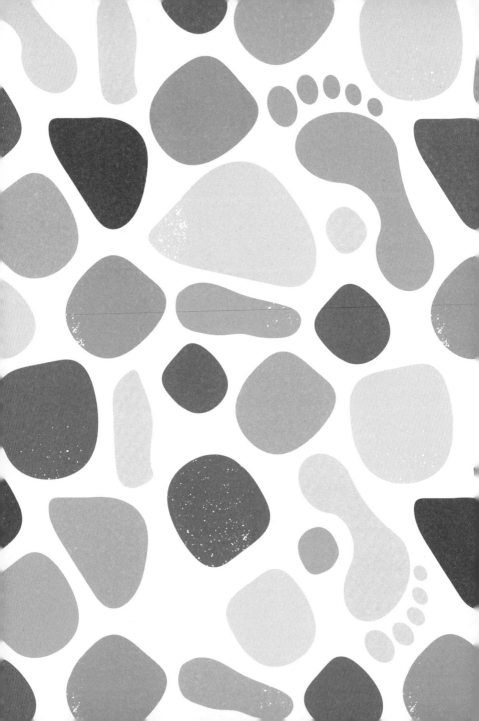

CHAPTER 12

HEEL PAIN

"My foot hurts first thing in the morning when I get out of bed." Does that sound familiar? Do you get up and your first step nearly knocks you to the floor? If so, you, like many others, may be suffering from plantar fasciitis. Heel pain is one of the most common complaints treated in a podiatry office, and more likely than not, plantar fasciitis is the culprit.

The plantar fascia is a strong band of tissue, similar to a thick ligament, that extends from the heel to the ball of the foot. There are three bands of the plantar fascia: a medial, central, and lateral band. The majority of people who suffer from plantar fasciitis get pain at the medial origin of the plantar fascia at the heel.

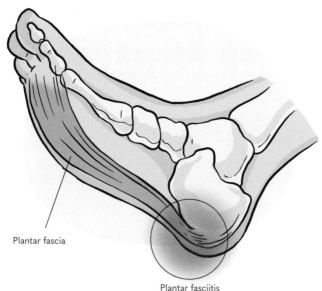

Plantar fascia

Plantar fasciitis

It's a common misconception that if you have plantar fasciitis, you must have heel spurs. The term "heel spur" is used quite often by other medical professionals because it is easily seen on an X-ray, making it a quick diagnosis for the patient. While heel spurs can be associated with plantar fasciitis, the pain that you are experiencing is actually not from the spur. The heel spur forms due to the inflammatory process that occurs at the plantar fascia for an overly tight band. As the plantar fasciitis becomes more chronic, the inflammatory cells cause a reactive process to the bone at the insertion site, causing more bone formation; hence, a spur develops. As the spur increases in size, the body has now created a shortened origin of the plantar fascia. This is the body's own way of trying to alleviate the pull from an overall tightened plantar fascia. The spur is parallel to the weight-bearing surface, pushing on any other soft tissue structures to cause pain. Patients can be pain-free with a large spur on an X-ray, or they can be in excruciating pain with no observable spur on an X-ray. The term heel spur syndrome is synonymous with plantar fasciitis.

So what causes plantar fasciitis? First and foremost, the lower extremities, from the hips down to the toes, act as a pulley and lever system. A fault in one part of the system can cause astronomical effects to the rest of the system. An overly tight hamstring, Achilles tendon, or plantar fascia can cause pain in secondary locations. When these soft tissue structures are tight, it increases the pull on the plantar fascia, causing the sharp heel pain associated with plantar fasciitis. This is important because if tightness is not addressed, whether it's secondary to your hamstring, Achilles tendon, plantar fascia, or all of the above, then the risk of pain recurrence is much higher, making for an unhappy patient.

One of the main causes for plantar fasciitis is lack of support and poor biomechanics of the foot. You may have heard the terms "pronation" and "overpronation." They are commonly used terms today when shopping for athletic shoes. Pronation is a normal part of your gait (walking), where the arch drops to the ground for shock absorption, momentarily allowing the heel to evert, and readying the foot for push-off. Over-pronation is when the heel stays in this everted position for too long in the gait cycle. This can cause excess stress to the joints and soft tissue in the foot, increasing the risk of developing plantar fasciitis. You don't necessarily have to be flat footed to get plantar fasciitis, though. People with high arches can also develop plantar fasciitis because of the tightness to the fascia and the lack of shock absorption associated with a high-arched foot. Without proper biomechanical support, regardless of your foot type, the likelihood of your heel pain going away and staying away drops significantly.

Heel pain can also present on the back of the heel, unlike plantar fasciitis, which is on the bottom of the heel. Achilles tendinitis is the most common cause for pain on the back of the heel. It may be localized to the heel or extend up the back of the ankle and leg as well. Some patients experience burning or tingling heel pain, which can be associated with nerve impingement or entrapment. Some patients have bursitis, which is usually directly in the center of the bottom of your heel. Finally, and much less common, is a stress fracture of the calcaneus, your heel bone. A test your practitioner may use to differentiate a stress fracture from plantar fasciitis is cupping the heel and pressing both sides. If this elicits pain, this is highly suspicious of a stress fracture, and further imaging may be necessary.

Confirming a case of plantar fasciitis is a relatively easy clinical diagnosis. While an X-ray may show a heel spur, you won't see the plantar fascia on it, because an X-ray does not visualize soft tissue well. An MRI may show thickening or swelling within the plantar fascia, as will an ultrasound, but ultimately a diagnosis is clinically based.

Typical complaints are "heel pain first thing in the morning," "sharp, stabbing pain in the bottom of my heel," and "it hurts when I get up from sitting." Acute plantar fasciitis hurts first thing in the morning and improves as the day progresses, while chronic plantar fasciitis hurts all the time. So the patient history and clinical workup are key to nailing down the diagnosis.

So, how do you treat plantar fasciitis? Keep in mind, it is not unusual to deal with plantar fasciitis for years. While we hope that the relief you get from treatment prevents plantar fasciitis from coming back, it is just not likely.

The two most basic ways of treating plantar fasciitis are stretching and icing. Stretching involves pulling your toes back toward your knee, elongating the plantar fascia and the Achilles tendon. Any type of calf or hamstring stretch is also helpful, as this lengthens the tendons that work in relation to one another. The goal of stretching is to improve the length of the plantar fascia, making it more flexible so it isn't as tight. This process of slowly elongating the plantar fascia alleviates inflammation at the insertion site on the heel, which eliminates pain.

Plantar fascia night splints are also recommended and are helpful for stretching. There are two types of night splints: one straps along the front of the leg, while the other straps along the back, like a boot. I usually recommend the splint along the back of your leg because it tends to give a better stretch. It is important to understand how to use a plantar fascia splint, because if worn incorrectly, it can cause more pressure on the ball of your foot, leading to numbness or tingling in your toes. Yes, you can sleep with the night splint, but it is bulky. I usually recommend wearing it for an hour each night before bedtime or while watching your favorite TV show.

Icing is recommended for ten to fifteen minutes, two to three times a day. Take a water bottle, freeze it, and roll it under your foot. It acts as an ice massage, and the firmness of the bottle kneads along the plantar fascia. If you don't have a frozen water bottle, use a tennis ball and roll it on the bottom of your foot for the same massaging effect. While stretching and icing by themselves may not completely alleviate the pain, it is imperative to utilize these techniques along with other treatments.

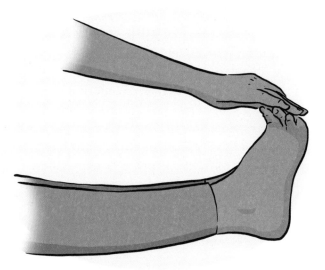

The most important treatment for plantar fasciitis, both acutely and long term, is using custom orthotics. If you forget everything else discussed in this chapter, remember this: custom orthotics are key to treating plantar fasciitis! Faulty biomechanics (how your foot functions during walking) are the main cause of pain associated with plantar fasciitis. Therefore, correcting the mechanics by improving the alignment of the foot is the best way to treat plantar fasciitis in the long term. Because orthotics play a key role in treatment, my patients always have a hard time with this next statement, but it is essential in treating acute plantar fasciitis: avoid walking barefoot. As a podiatrist based in Florida, I understand this is a tough task for my patients. But as I tell them, avoiding barefoot walking (or at least minimizing it) must play a part in the treatment plan to improve heel pain.

Sometimes an orthotic alone may not alleviate plantar fasciitis pain, but that doesn't mean the orthotics aren't working. Orthotics are an essential item to use with other modalities of treatment. There are many types of generic over-the-counter inserts that can be quite costly. Even though they are more accessible, save your money and invest in custom orthotics. They will be made for you and last longer. Do not buy orthotics from anyone other than a podiatrist. Don't buy them at a shoe store. Don't buy them at a carnival pop-up tent. Don't buy them on a cruise. A podiatrist is the only person who truly understands the dynamics and biomechanics of your foot to correctly make an orthotic for you. Our training in biomechanics excels far beyond any course taken over the weekend by a hired employee to sell you inserts at a store. You wouldn't buy your eyeglasses from a vendor at a flea market. So don't buy your orthotics there either. If you are scanned for orthotics at a shoe store and then handed an "orthotic" off a shelf, it is not a custom orthotic. Shoe stores tend to charge more, and you get less. When a custom orthotic is made, your foot must be held in a neutral position, and adjustments must be made to the orthotic to accommodate for any pathology we may note. If you stand on a scanning pad without someone holding your foot in a neutral position, you are essentially making a misaligned insert for your foot. Unfortunately, I see it time and time again. Patients spend hundreds of dollars on "custom" orthotics from a shoe store, only to find out they work better as a bookmark than as a steady support for your body. Your feet are the foundation of your body; they need professional support.

Anti-inflammatory medications are the next stalwart in alleviating plantar fasciitis pain. As we discussed above, if your feet hurt, even with your custom orthotics, it's not because the orthotics are not working; you may just need an anti-inflammatory added to the treatment plan. The most effective way to decrease plantar fasciitis pain is with a cortisone injection. Typically, you can have up to three cortisone injections in a year without any major side effects. Oral anti-inflammatories or topicals are also helpful; they are just not as long lasting as an injection and may not be as effective because of the difficulty in getting the medication to such a small, relatively minimally vascular area of the foot. An injection by itself, without other treatments such as stretching and custom orthotics, is a band-aid effect. An injection along with these other forms of treatment acts synergistically, optimizing the patient's satisfaction.

Regenerative medicine is becoming increasingly popular for treating chronic plantar fasciitis. In some patients, chronic plantar fasciitis has been present for months to years. It does not respond to standard treatment, and prior to regenerative medicine, many patients succumbed to surgery for pain relief. Treatment options for chronic plantar fasciitis (also called plantar fasciosis) include extracorporeal shock wave therapy; cold laser treatments, with or without electric stimulation; platelet-rich plasma injections (PRP); and stem cell injections. The goal of all of these modalities is to increase or create an inflammatory response in an otherwise chronic, dormant area of pain; to trigger the body to start the healing cascade of events by the immune system. Personally, I've had a great deal of success with shockwave therapy, cold laser treatments, and PRP.

The recovery process for these modalities varies, since they utilize your own body to heal the area of interest. Shock wave and laser treatments typically don't require any downtime, while PRP and stem cell injections include wearing a walking boot for a couple of weeks afterward. Most of these modalities are not covered by insurance and can be costly, but they are a great alternative to surgery. Following the completion of these treatments, you will want to be sure you are in proper orthotics and, again, performing stretching exercises to maintain a pain-free foot. Sometimes physical therapy is warranted because the tightness of the plantar fascia may still be present, which is a reason plantar fasciitis may have started in the first place.

The final option for chronic plantar fasciitis is a plantar fasciotomy. This involves surgically cutting a part of the band of the plantar fascia to release it. Surgical release allows the plantar fascia to heal in an elongated, stretched position. This surgery can be done in-office or in a surgery center with sedation. After surgery, a walking boot is required for a couple of weeks until the stitches are removed. One of the biggest concerns with a plantar fasciotomy is recurrence of pain or pain that has transferred to another spot on the bottom of the heel.

Plantar fasciitis is one of the most common problems we face in our profession and can be stubborn to treat. Some people can get complete resolution of symptoms just by stretching and icing, while others do all the options listed above and still can't get relief. The same protocol doesn't work for everyone when it comes to treating plantar fasciitis; however, staying consistent and compliant with the treatments your podiatrist provides for you is the best way to get rid of your heel pain.

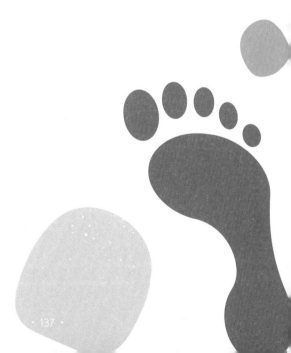

FAQs

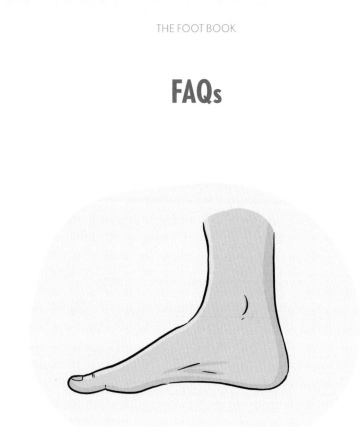

Why do the bottom of my heels hurt first thing in the morning?

When you're sleeping, your plantar fascia shortens and tightens because it is in a relaxed position. When you get out of bed and step down in the morning, it causes a sudden pull or strain of the plantar fascia, which immediately leads to the pain.

Is it OK to walk around barefoot or wear flip-flops all the time?

No. While you are treating plantar fasciitis, you want to avoid being barefoot or wearing unsupportive shoes at all costs. Wear house shoes when walking in your home and use supportive shoes with custom orthotics.

Will my heel spur go away?

No, but heel spurs on the bottom of the heel do not cause pain. The pain is originating from inflammation of the plantar fascia. Surgically removing the heel spur and not treating the plantar fascia will ultimately lead to failure in treatment.

Should I just buy inserts at the shoe store?

Before buying inserts at the shoe store, I would make an appointment with your podiatrist to discuss custom orthotics. The shoe store inserts are not custom made for you.

Will plantar fasciitis ever go away?

Yes, it will. You must remain consistent and compliant with treatment, but it can go away. How long will it take? Everyone is different.

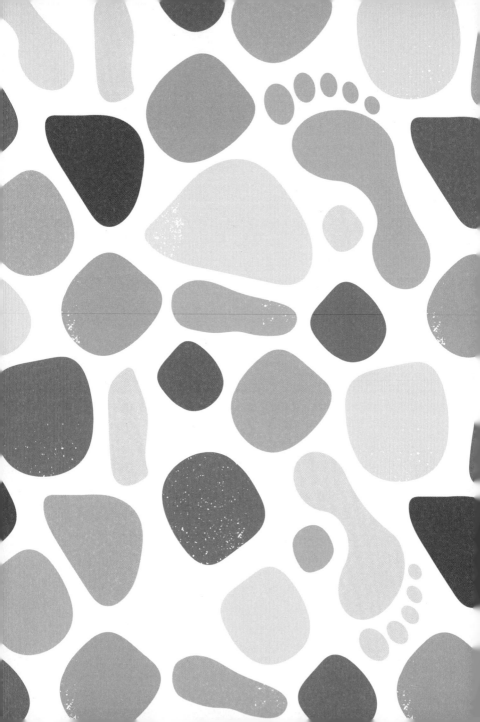

CHAPTER 13

FLATFEET AND HIGH ARCHES

There are three common foot types: a neutral foot, a high-arch foot, and a flat foot. While a neutral foot type is considered "normal," common foot ailments can manifest in a neutral foot just as easily as in someone with an "abnormal" foot type. The two other foot types, flat foot and high-arch (cavus) foot, present with differing complaints.

A high-arch foot, or cavus foot, is less common compared to a flatfoot deformity; however, it is worth discussing, as people with a cavus foot structure have a difficult foot type to treat. There are several different etiologies for cavus foot structure. One of the most common reasons a person may have a cavus foot is from an underlying neurological condition. Charcot-Marie-Tooth disease, a history of strokes, and cerebral palsy are common neurological conditions associated with cavus foot deformity. Other times it can simply be an inherited foot type without explanation. Depending on the severity of the cavus foot deformity, the main complaints are ankle sprains, pain on top of the arch, hammertoe deformities, and pain on the outside of the foot. Ankle sprains are common with a cavus foot type, because there is less surface area on the bottom of the foot contacting the ground. More ground contact on the outside of the foot and less contact of the arch make it easier for a patient's foot to twist inward inadvertently, causing an ankle sprain. Pain can also be associated with the top of the arch, due to irritation of the nerves (neuritis) on top of the foot when in contact with restrictive shoe gear. Allotment of more flexible uppers helps reduce neuritis in patients with a cavus foot. Hammertoe deformities (see Chapter 4) can develop from faulty biomechanics associated with a cavus foot. It is a commonly heard complaint to experience pain on the outside of the foot in patients with a cavus foot type. This is simply due to the arch not contacting the ground during walking, decreasing the ability to absorb shock in the foot. Without proper shock absorption, the foot acts as a rigid lever and will hit the ground heavily from heel strike to toe off.

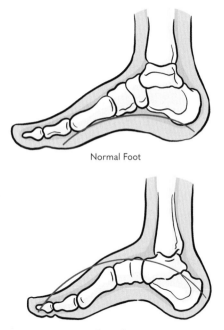

Normal Foot

Cavus Foot

Treatment options for cavus feet are available through conservative and surgical measures. Conservative treatments will assist in the reduction of symptoms but will not decrease the arch height or "cure" a cavus foot type. Custom orthotics are an absolute necessity in this population of patients, simply due to off-the-shelf inserts being incapable of contacting the high arch associated with a cavus foot. There are surgical procedures to correct a cavus foot. Usually, a combination of surgical procedures with osteotomies (cut in the bone) and soft tissue procedures, such as tendon transfers, is performed to rebalance the mechanics of the foot. The recovery is approximately six to eight weeks, non-weight-bearing to partial weight bearing in a cast or boot, depending on the surgeon's preference. If you are considering surgical intervention, a thorough physical exam and evaluation should be performed with your surgeon to determine which procedures are right for your foot.

Another common foot type is a flat foot. Flatfoot is a condition that has other names associated with it, such as "fallen arches" and "overpronation." Regardless of which term you use, it is the complaint of pain essentially originating from the collapse of the arch.

There are several causes for flatfoot deformity; however, the most prevalent cause is genetics. If your family has a history of flatfeet, you are more prone to developing flatfeet as well. So, check out your parents' and grandparents' feet the next time you see them. Chances are your feet will look like theirs as well.

Another cause for flatfeet is a condition called tarsal coalition. A tarsal coalition occurs at birth when two bones in your foot merge and fuse together, bridging over a joint and causing the joint to not move. Not only does this cause flatfoot, but it can also cause a severe lack of motion throughout the foot.

Another etiology for flatfeet is injury to the posterior tibial tendon, which is the primary tendon that helps support the arch.

Finally, those with trisomy genetic disorders such as Down syndrome commonly have flatfeet and require treatment to improve the ability to ambulate with less pain.

If you have flatfeet, the deformity usually originates from more than a sagittal drop in the arch. It is a multiplanar deformity, meaning the flat foot can develop in up to three planes: the sagittal plane, the frontal plane, and the transverse plane. It is important to know which plane the flat foot is predominantly affected by, because it helps the physician tailor your treatment if surgical intervention is necessary.

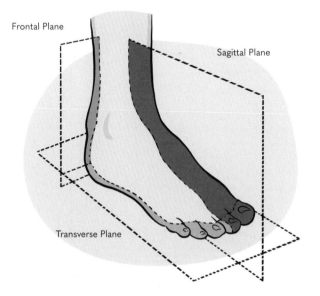

How do you diagnose flatfeet, other than simply by looking at the foot? X-rays are a normal part of the protocol for workup of a flat foot. They can offer the provider useful information with regard to the effect a flat foot has had on the joints and whether a tarsal coalition is present. There are specific angles of the foot bones that a podiatrist looks at to help determine the severity of flatfoot as well. Obviously, examining the foot can present a clear clinical picture as to whether you have flatfoot, but X-rays can provide additional details that are essential to treatment plans.

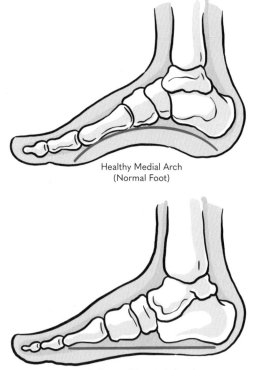

Healthy Medial Arch
(Normal Foot)

Collapse of the Medial Arch
(Flat Foot)

Common areas associated with flatfoot pain include the top of the foot, the outside of the ankle, the Achilles, or the plantar fascia. Certain motions, including side-to-side motions of your heel and up-and-down motions of your ankle, can elicit pain in a flatfoot deformity. Flatfeet can also affect joints in other areas besides the joints in your foot, including the ankles, knees, and hips.

There are two types of flatfeet: rigid and flexible. It is important that your podiatrist determines your type in order to best differentiate and outline treatment options.

Rigid flatfeet may be caused by arthritis, birth defects, or tarsal coalitions. A rigid deformity indicates that when the physician tries to recreate your arch, he or she cannot, due to a bony block preventing motion. While rigid flatfeet tends to be more resistant to conservative treatments, nonsurgical treatment should still be attempted.

Flexible flatfeet is both a bony and soft tissue deformity, and it allows the arch to be recreated by the physician when manipulated on exam. A flexible deformity tends to respond better to conservative treatment, and it is initiated on the initial presentation.

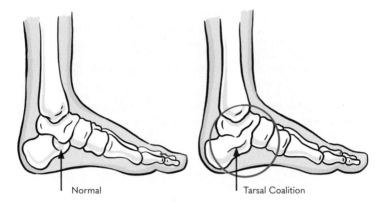

Normal   Tarsal Coalition

If your flatfoot is rigid due to arthritis, birth defects, or
tarsal coalitions as discussed above, I'd recommend trying
conservative care first, such as injections, custom orthotics,
and bracing; however, surgical intervention is typically
required at some point in the patient's lifetime. Though performing isolated injections in the affected foot joint may be
helpful, these benefits are usually short lived. Another option
is a custom-made orthotic. An orthotic used for rigid flatfoot
is called an accommodative orthotic. The primary goal of an
accommodative orthotic is to support the foot, preventing
excess motion to improve pain. If, however, the options listed
above fail, then surgical intervention is typically warranted.
If you have a tarsal coalition, the coalition or bony bridge
could be resected to try to restore the motion; however,
the risk of recurrence is high, meaning that the bony bridge
could recur between the two joints. The primary surgical
treatment for rigid flatfoot is an arthrodesis. This means that
the affected joints are fused together, after placing the foot
in a neutral position that allows for reformation of the arch.
Usually, healthy patients require eight weeks for healing from

the surgery. The complications associated with this procedure include infection, malunion (fused in the incorrect position) or nonunion (does not fuse), and recurrence of pain.

If you have flexible flatfoot, then your chances of conservative care being successful are much higher than those with rigid flatfoot. Localized cortisone injections in conjunction with a custom orthotic are much more likely to result in resolution of pain than attempting those treatments as isolated procedures. When the custom orthotic is made for flexible flatfoot, your foot is held in a corrected position to assure the orthotic holds you there long term. An orthotic is not something you wear for a short period of time to recreate the arch permanently. An orthotic is a lifelong treatment. There are also surgical treatments generally termed "flatfoot reconstructions." This type of surgery utilizes a combination of bone cuts and soft tissue procedures (ligament repairs or tendon transfers) to recreate the arch while leaving the joints intact, thereby sustaining motion to the foot. The combined procedures aim to correct the flat foot in multiple planes, since it is typically a multiplanar deformity. Again, a physician must evaluate which planes are affected in order to determine the necessary procedures. The recovery for these procedures is approximately six to eight weeks non-weight-bearing in a cast or immobilization boot. Complications are similar to those listed above for an arthrodesis, including but not limited to infection, recurrence of flatfoot, or continued pain.

Having flatfeet, whether flexible or rigid, doesn't necessarily mean you're destined for surgery. Always be sure to attempt conservative care first before jumping into surgery. Orthotics are a mainstay treatment for flatfeet and should always be utilized even when surgery is performed. Contact your doctor for a consultation if you have painful flat feet that require further care.

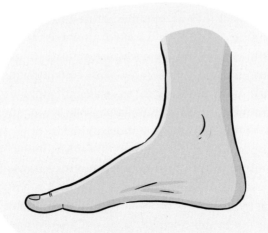

FAQs

Is it normal for kids to be flat footed?

Yes, it is. Arch formation begins to occur when children develop a normal gait as they develop.

Can flatfeet be corrected?

Yes. Flexible flatfeet can be corrected with orthotics or surgery, while rigid flatfeet can only be fully corrected with surgery.

Can flatfeet lead to any other problems?

Absolutely. Having flatfeet can lead to pain in your ankles, knees, hips, or back.

Should I try generic inserts to help my flatfoot pain?

I would not. If you are flat footed, it is advisable to have orthotics custom made by a podiatrist who can correctly manipulate your foot and hold it in a neutral position to create your custom orthotics.

Do you always have pain with flatfeet?

No. You can be flat footed and have no pain, especially in adolescence or early adulthood. Soft tissues tend to adapt easier to abnormalities when we are younger. However, as the aging process occurs, our soft tissue is less adaptable and may not be able to compensate as well; therefore, pain will occur. Some of it depends on luck, but more commonly it depends on your activity level.

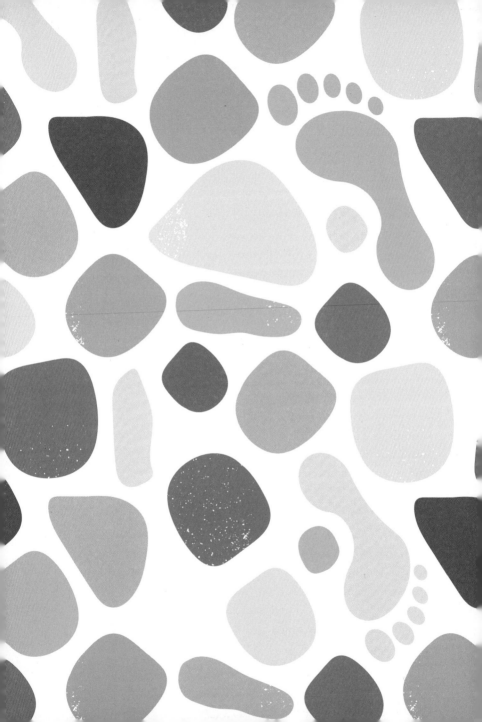

CHAPTER 14

ARCH PAIN

While "arch pain" can be understood as a vague term, and can sometimes be confused with plantar fasciitis, it is a definitive issue unique from other foot problems.

Arch pain is associated with the posterior tibial tendon (also called the PT tendon). This tendon inserts in the arch, and when it is inflamed or not functioning correctly, it can cause arch pain as well as pain along the side of your ankle. When the PT tendon is inflamed, it is called posterior tibial tendinitis. When the PT tendon is not working properly, the condition is called posterior tibial tendon dysfunction (PTTD).

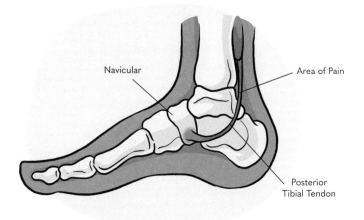

Common complaints that are associated with PTTD are flattening of the arch, pain along the side of the ankle, pain when raising up on your toes, or a noticeable bump forming along the side of the arch. These specific clinical findings will help your podiatrist differentiate PTTD from plantar fasciitis. When being examined in the office, you may have discomfort and pain behind your ankle bone along the inside of your ankle. Since the tendon courses around the leg, extending to the foot, it is not uncommon to experience symptoms along the foot and ankle. The prominent bump on the inside of your arch is the navicular bone, where the tendon inserts in your foot. A well-trained provider will likely ask you to perform a heel raise test (either a single or double heel raise) to evaluate how well or how poorly the tendon is functioning, as well as whether the test elicits pain.

The main cause of PTTD is the tendon fatiguing from an over-pronating foot. As discussed in the chapter about flatfeet (see Chapter 13), overpronation causes the heel to evert, which places increased strain along the PT tendon at the arch. When a person with flatfoot walks, the arch collapses, placing more strain on the PT tendon. This imbalance of force and pull causes the tendon to become inflamed and painful. Eventually, the tendon can become so overworked from the abnormal pull in an overpronated foot that the tendon will eventually fatigue and stop working. This is when the patient sees a dramatic collapse in the arch, causing severe PTTD.

Another cause of PTTD is being born with an os tibiale externum (OTE), which is an accessory bone that develops near, or at the prominent portion of, the navicular bone. Not only does OTE cause a large bump on the inside of the arch, creating a cosmetic issue, it can cause shearing force along the posterior tibial tendon with everyday walking or exercise. The constant shearing force can cause long-term pain, but very rarely will lead to a rupture. While rupturing the PT tendon is unusual, it can occur. In the case of an acute rupture, the

PT tendon is strained to the extreme, pulling the tendon off of the insertion on the navicular bone and, typically, pulling off a piece of the bone with it. This traumatic incident causes an immediate, profound collapse of the arch and should be evaluated immediately.

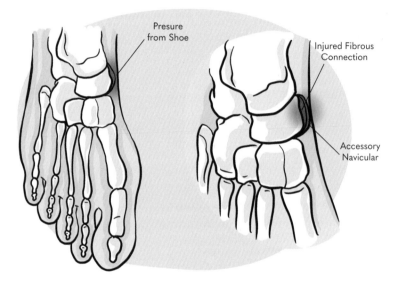

Presure from Shoe

Injured Fibrous Connection

Accessory Navicular

So what can be done to alleviate your pain? If you are dealing with acute pain associated with PT tendinitis, icing, anti-inflammatories, and stretches are helpful for building up strength and reducing inflammation of the tendon. I typically tell my patients to spell out the alphabet with their foot when exercising. These treatment tips tend to work when you have tendinitis associated with overexercising or walking all day in an amusement park. Now while these treatment options will help to improve pain and strength, finding stability and support is important for long-term treatment goals.

Custom orthotics and shoe gear are imperative to help alleviate PT tendon pain and prevent it from coming back. If pain persists after attempting the options mentioned above, physical therapy may be a helpful way to improve strength and stability in the PT tendon. For chronic PTTD, an immobilization walking boot may be issued to the patient, to allow the tendon to rest and reduce abnormal pressure during gait. Typically, we place patients in a walking boot for four to six weeks, depending on how long the tendon has been chronically injured. By alleviating the pressure on the tendon, the goal is to reduce inflammation, which will reduce pain. Finally, regenerative medicine options, such as laser treatment, shock wave therapy, and platelet-rich plasma (PRP) injections, show promising data about relieving the pain associated with chronic PTTD. As discussed in previous chapters, these modalities work by signaling regenerating cells in your body to be triggered and allowing the body to heal itself. These modalities are not typically covered by insurance and are not provided by all doctors. So check with your provider to see if he or she has regenerative medicine services in-office.

If conservative treatments fail to alleviate your PT tendon pain, an MRI may be ordered to provide more detailed imaging, evaluating for a tear or degenerative qualities of the tendon. This is important to establish, especially if you are considering surgery to help repair the tendon or utilize it for reconstructive procedures for the arch.

If the MRI reveals tearing of the PT tendon or thickening of the tendon, then a primary surgical repair is necessary. A tear in the tendon must be debrided or debulked, to get rid of the inflammatory tissue and to expose the solid healthy tissue surrounding it. If the PT tendon is thickened with fatty tendon substitute, a common reaction to chronically injured tissue, then it is removed, leaving only a healthy, functional tendon. A nonabsorbable suture is then used to tubularize (wrap around) the tendon to help reinforce and strengthen it, reducing the risk of further degenerative changes. Occasionally a cadaveric or biologic graft is sutured into the tendon to provide structural reinforcement. The recovery is typically six to eight weeks in a walking boot, partial to non-weight-bearing.

If the MRI shows thickening of the tendon at the insertion point and an os tibiale externum (accessory bone) is present, then a different surgical procedure may be required than those listed above. If the accessory bone or a large bony prominence is appreciated on the navicular bone (primary bone the PT tendon inserts), then the tendon is dissected and removed from the insertion point on the bone and reflected to expose the accessory bone or the large bony prominence. Then the os tibiale externum is excised, or a bone cut is made to remove the large bony prominence. The tendon is then reapproximated and anchored back to the bone with soft tissue anchors. This not only removes the unsightly or painful bump on the side of the arch, but it also provides a better form of leverage for the PT tendon, therefore improving its function. The recovery for this procedure is approximately six to eight weeks, non-weight-bearing in an immobilization boot. The possible complications associated with this procedure are rupturing the tendon, tendon weakness, chronic pain, and swelling.

Finally, if the pain to the arch and tendon is secondary to the functionality of the foot, such as that of a flat foot, then the procedure will follow that of the ones discussed in detail in Chapter 13. These procedures typically involve both tendon and bone work to help realign the foot and arch, and recovery is about six to eight weeks for this as well.

So, while arch pain is commonly confused with plantar fasciitis, it is almost always a distinctive problem that should be addressed on a patient-by-patient basis. Being sure to support the foot properly with an orthotic and improve the strength and inflammation of the tendon are imperative in a successful recovery.

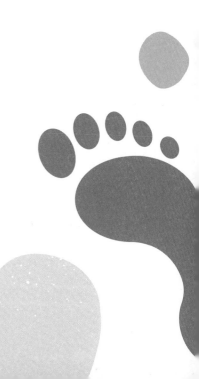

FAQs

What is the bump on the side of my foot?

This bump is part of a bone called the navicular. It is the bone that the majority of the PT tendon inserts on, which is the primary tendon that supports the arch. When associated with pain, it usually has an excess bony growth or an accessory bone called an os tibiale externum that is identified on a foot X-ray.

Does my arch pain have anything to do with being flat-footed?

Yes. The more your foot pronates, the more strain is placed on the PT tendon, causing pain along the arch extending up to the ankle.

My arch doesn't hurt. It feels closer to the side of my ankle. Could that be related to my arch pain?

Yes. The tendon that inserts on your arch extends up past your ankle and originates deep in your leg.

Do I need surgery if my tendon is torn?

No, not necessarily. It is still recommended to try conservative care, whether it is immobilization or regenerative medicine, prior to surgical intervention. If either of these methods fails, then your podiatrist should talk to you about surgical repair of the tendon.

Why does it hurt when I go up steps or push up on my toes?

The main reason is because the PT tendon contracts and causes rubbing and friction at the insertion site on the navicular bone, leading to constant pain and inflammation.

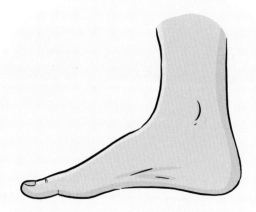

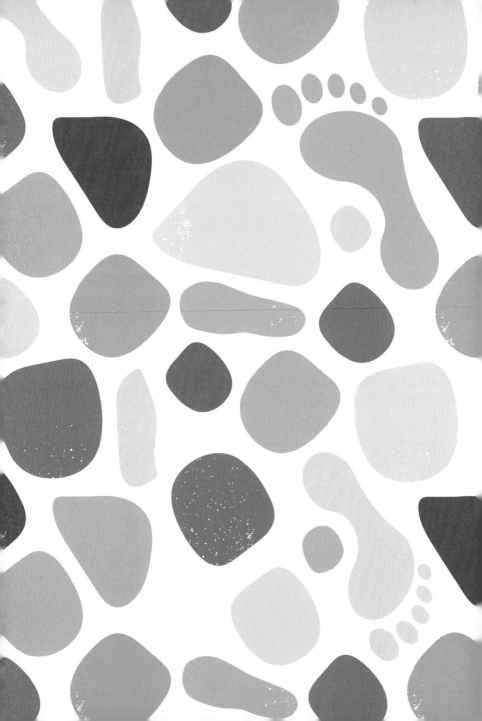

CHAPTER 15

ACHILLES TENDINITIS

Achilles tendinitis is the other type of heel pain that podiatrists commonly have described to them by patients. Most people think of plantar fasciitis as the culprit for heel pain; however, Achilles tendinitis can present with pain in the heel as well.

The Achilles is the strongest tendon in your body. It originates from the calf muscles called the gastrocnemius and soleus muscles, and inserts distally into the back of your heel. When the Achilles tendon contracts, it pulls your foot down (plantar flexes) and helps you push off when walking. The Achilles tendon fibers are interconnected with the plantar fascia in the heel. The Achilles is also interconnected to the hamstring group of muscles in the thigh. This interconnected relationship explains why one muscle group in the lower extremity can indirectly affect another. They are all working together in a lever system. When one part of the lever is not working optimally, the rest of the mechanics are affected. Another important part of the Achilles tendon anatomy is called the watershed area. It is located approximately four to six centimeters above the heel. It's the most palpable part of the Achilles tendon, commonly called the "heel cord." The watershed area has the least amount of blood flow to the Achilles tendon, increasing the risk for injury.

As we discussed with plantar fasciitis (see Chapter 12), over time a tight Achilles tendon can lead to a spur developing on the back of the heel. Unlike plantar fasciitis, the spur at the attachment site of the Achilles can actually cause pain due to its location. As the tight Achilles tendon contracts and pulls at the insertion site, inflammation will begin to occur along

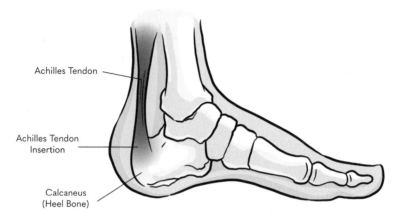

the back of the heel, which causes the spur to form. Most commonly, the initial pain is associated with the bone spur due to shoe irritation. Then as the spur enlarges, pain will be associated with direct palpation.

Clinically, when someone presents with Achilles tendon pain, they commonly report pain on the back of the heel. Other symptoms include tightness in the back of the leg; a large, prominent bump that is rubbing in shoes; or pain when lying in bed, because of direct pressure to the back of the heel. Swelling goes hand in hand with the bump on the back of the heel. The bump you see is typically a spur or calcification of the underlying bone, leading to thickening (or tendinopathy) of the Achilles. It is not uncommon to develop bursitis in this area as well, which causes swelling associated with the bone spur. A telltale sign can be when the patient complains of pain at the back of the heel while sitting in a chair or lying in bed. Basically, any activity that puts pressure on the back of the heel where the spur is directly located will elicit pain.

How do you get Achilles tendinitis? Ultimately it comes down to biomechanics. A tight hamstring and/or calf muscle can cause a disruption in the normal mechanics of the Achilles tendon, placing excess strain on the tendon. Flatfoot or a high-arch foot can place more stress on the Achilles tendon as well. This constant pulling leads to a sharp pain at the back of the heel. Women who regularly wear high-heel shoes are more prone to Achilles tendinitis. Consistently wearing high heels can lead to acquired equinus. Equinus is a term for decreased motion at the ankle joint due to tightness of the Achilles tendon. Acquired equinus means that your Achilles tendon shortens over time because of the shortened position it is constantly in, unlike congenital equinus, which is a shortened Achilles tendon from birth. Wearing heels regularly and not stretching properly after exercise are a couple of examples of how the tendon can shorten over time, causing acquired equinus. In fact, many patients with equinus complain of more pain in flat shoes than heels, because the flat shoe causes too much pull on the Achilles tendon, eliciting pain.

So, you know you have a spur. Does that mean you will experience pain? No, it does not. You can have a spur or calcification on the heel and still be pain-free. The development of a heel spur does, however, alter the mechanics of the Achilles tendon, increasing the risk of a strain or rupture to the tendon. The Achilles is already tight, and the spur can cause an additional shearing effect to the fibers of the tendon inserting on the bone, increasing the risk of tearing. You may have heard the term "weekend warrior." This is a common term used for middle-aged men who play basketball on the weekend but lead a fairly sedentary lifestyle during the week.

During a weekend game, overexertion of the tendon occurs, which consequently could lead to a loud pop that indicates a rupture. The most common area of the Achilles tendon to rupture with this sort of activity is the "watershed area" discussed earlier. In older patients, or geriatric populations, Achilles rupture is more common at the insertional site on the bone, where the fibers are weaker at the attachment.

How do you fix a spur with Achilles tendinitis? Some of the most basic treatment methods include icing and stretching. Any type of ankle joint range-of-motion exercises will help to improve the tightness of the Achilles tendon. Stretching two to three times a day is beneficial to produce lengthening over time to the tendon. Icing for ten to fifteen minutes a day and taking anti-inflammatories such as ibuprofen or Motrin are recommended treatments, as with any other form of tendinitis. The most utilized anti-inflammatory medication is a prepackaged dosed steroid taken for six days.

Receiving a cortisone injection at or near the Achilles tendon is not recommended because it could cause a spontaneous rupture of the tendon.

Custom orthotics with a small lift at the heel are another important conservative treatment option for Achilles tendinitis. An abnormal strain is placed on the Achilles tendon with overpronation, which will cause consistent pain to the heel. Properly supporting your arch and realigning the foot into a more neutral position during gait is a good way to stop the biomechanical fault that occurs with overpronation. This, in turn, alleviates stress from the Achilles tendon to reduce pain.

If the above-mentioned treatments have been unsuccessful, a referral to physical therapy can be extremely helpful toward improving the strength, stability, and range of motion of the Achilles tendon. More important, physical therapy can work on your entire lower extremity and home in on the primary problem, whether it is your hamstring, calf, or plantar fascia.

An alternative to physical therapy is immobilization in a walking boot. The walking boot locks your foot and ankle at ninety degrees to prevent motion at the Achilles, allowing it to rest fully and ultimately heal itself. The average period for immobilization is around four to six weeks, but this time frame can vary from patient to patient.

The last conservative option is regenerative medicine. This includes laser treatments, shockwave treatments, and platelet-rich plasma (PRP). As mentioned in other chapters, these modalities are not typically covered by insurance, but they can be highly effective in pain reduction and regeneration of tissue that has been chronically torn. Both shockwave and laser treatments require, on average, three to six treatments for normal results. PRP is one of the regenerative treatment options that my office uses as a first-line treatment because the results are typically satisfactory for patients with minimal comorbidities. The postoperative recovery requires immobilization in a walking boot for two weeks to allow for the tissue to begin the regeneration process. In my opinion, PRP is the best treatment for Achilles tendinitis with an accompanying spur, and should be discussed with patients early in the treatment process.

If all else fails, surgical intervention is warranted. Keep in mind that if you do suffer from an acute Achilles rupture, then immediate repair is recommended. The procedure entails detaching the Achilles tendon to expose the prominent bone spur. The bone spur is removed, and the Achilles tendon is anchored back to the bone and secured in place with bone anchors. If there is thickening of the Achilles from chronic inflammation, it is usually debulked to remove any inflamed tissue. Sometimes a biologic graft may be used to reinforce the Achilles and aid in better healing overall. The aftercare for a bone spur removal with reattachment of the Achilles tendon is typically non-weight-bearing in a walking boot or cast for six to eight weeks. Following this period of no weight, the patient is then transitioned to weight bearing in a walking boot for an additional one to two weeks, and finally to regular supportive tennis shoes. It is a long process, but one that usually has successful results. Possible complications include swelling, nerve pain, postoperative tightness of the Achilles tendon, and infection. Ensuring that you have the ability to stay off your foot during the healing process is essential, as this procedure has a high risk of rupture with early weight bearing to the surgical foot.

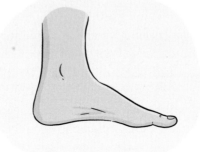

FAQs

How did I develop a spur?

The constant pulling of a tight Achilles tendon on the bone will cause inflammation to develop, therefore causing bone to react and enlarge.

Am I at an increased risk of rupturing my Achilles if there is a bone spur present?

Yes, in certain circumstances. If you are a middle-aged, sedentary individual who performs rigorous activities casually a few times a week, you are at a higher risk of injury because your body is not used to the activity level you are performing. Warming up your muscles prior to the activity and proper stretching can reduce the risk of injury.

What is the best nonoperative treatment?

In my opinion, platelet-rich plasma is the most successful and quickest treatment to alleviate Achilles tendinitis, in combination with immobilization in a walking boot.

Will the spur go away without surgery?

No. The pain may go away without surgery; however, the only way to remove the spur is surgical excision.

What is the bump on the back of my heel?

The bump is usually the prominent spur with subsequent thickening of the Achilles. You will also get localized swelling called bursitis from the pain and irritation of the Achilles tendon rubbing on shoe gear.

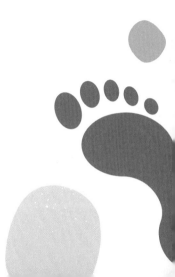

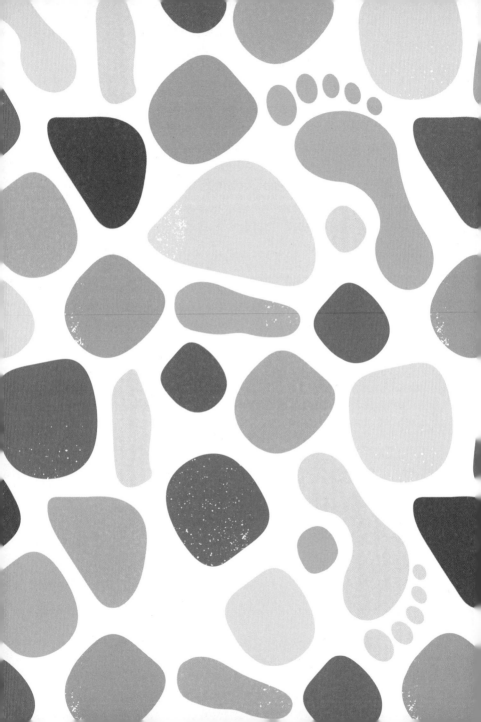

CHAPTER 16

ARTHRITIS

There are many arthritic conditions that a person can suffer from throughout the body; however, this chapter will examine those most commonly encountered in the foot and ankle. Psoriatic arthritis, rheumatoid arthritis, and osteoarthritis (degenerative joint disease) will be discussed in depth. Gout is also a common type of arthritis; however, please refer to Chapter 9, which discusses gout manifestations in the foot and ankle.

Psoriatic Arthritis

Psoriatic arthritis is an inflammatory arthritis found in the smaller joints of the foot. Psoriatic arthritis is not as well understood by the general public in comparison to some other arthritides; however, it is becoming a mainstream topic in medicine, with promising medications more readily available. Psoriatic arthritis is an autoimmune disease associated with psoriasis that affects the hand and foot joints. The typical skin plaques associated with psoriasis might develop, but joint pain and swelling do not occur. All patients who have psoriasis do not have psoriatic arthritis. In fact, medical literature suggests that psoriatic arthritis only affects 7 to 26 percent of psoriasis patients. All psoriatic arthritis patients, however, have psoriasis. Having the textbook skin plaques associated with psoriasis does not always precede arthritic changes either, which can make the diagnosis difficult.

Swelling, redness, and warmth to the touch of the small joints of the toes is typically the initial presentation of psoriatic arthritis. It can affect one toe or multiple toes on the same foot, or both feet. The presentation of swelling, redness, and warmth to the toes is commonly described as "sausage digits." As the disease itself progresses, the joint can become significantly arthritic, which can lead to loss of motion, stiffness, and increased pain in the joint. Changes to the toenail on the affected digit may also present as small pits or ridges on the nail. Although this may be cosmetically displeasing, pain or skin complications are usually absent. Psoriatic arthritis can affect areas other than the toes as well. It can also cause irritation or thickening at the insertion of the Achilles tendon and/or plantar fascia. This, in turn, can cause chronic plantar fasciitis and Achilles tendinitis. For more information on these conditions, please see the Chapters 12 and 15, which are dedicated to these conditions.

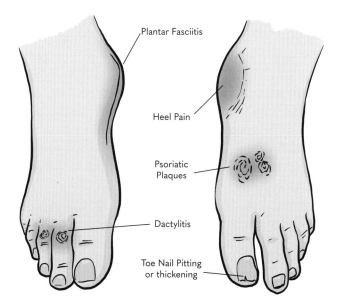

Plantar Fasciitis

Heel Pain

Psoriatic Plaques

Dactylitis

Toe Nail Pitting or thickening

The exact cause of psoriatic arthritis is unknown; however, a family history may increase your risk or predispose you to developing psoriatic arthritis. Keep in mind that psoriasis is a multisystem disease process. This discussion is solely about the arthritic component and how it pertains to the feet. Diagnosis can be difficult since there isn't a quick test or study available to positively diagnose psoriatic arthritis. A rheumatology lab panel is performed, with blood tests such as HLA and rheumatoid factor being helpful indicators to lead to or eliminate psoriatic arthritis as a diagnosis.

Just as with any autoimmune disease, early detection is essential to control or slow the progression of long-term effects associated with psoriatic arthritis. Medication management for psoriatic arthritis is usually performed by a rheumatologist; however, a multidisciplinary team approach is essential to assist with the systemic issues associated with this particular autoimmune disease.

Oral medications such as anti-inflammatories or disease-modifying anti-rheumatic drugs are treatments utilized for pain relief and slowing the progression of the disease. Local cortisone injections are also good treatment options available to help alleviate the pain and swelling from an acute flare-up of a psoriatic arthritis joint.

If the joint has progressed to a point where medications or injections are not sufficient enough to reduce pain, then surgical intervention may be warranted. Since psoriatic arthritis attacks the small joints of the toes, treatments would be similar to that of a hammertoe. Performing an arthroplasty, which involves removing part of the joint to alleviate the pain and irritation, is a possibility. You could expect about a two-week recovery period for this treatment. The other option is an arthrodesis, which is fusing the affected joint so it doesn't move anymore, therefore alleviating the pain. The recovery for a procedure like this is around four to six weeks. Patients are usually encouraged to pursue arthrodesis, as this procedure is less likely to have recurrent symptoms of psoriatic "flare-ups," since the joint is fused.

Rheumatoid Arthritis

Rheumatoid arthritis (RA) is the more commonly known arthritis among the general population. RA is typically hereditary in nature, and, similar to psoriatic arthritis, it is an autoimmune disease that affects multiple systems in the body.

RA is considered polyarticular, meaning it affects multiple joints, and is usually symmetrical, affecting the hands and/or feet. Early symptoms include swelling, pain, and redness to the knuckles in the hands and feet. The most common joints affected in the feet are the metatarsophalangeal joints. As the disease progresses, deviation of the toes occurs, causing the toes to direct outward or lateralize. It can also affect the smaller joints in the toes, which can lead to hammertoe contractures and pain. RA can lead to chronic arthritic changes to the affected joints, resulting in stiffness and pain. In fact, a very consistent finding with RA is pain and stiffness for about an hour after waking up from a night of sleep. Elderly patients with RA tend to have pain in their feet because of the combination of foot deformities associated with RA, in conjunction with atrophy of the fat pad from the natural aging process. The increased pressure on the ball of the foot or the arch can also lead to rheumatoid nodules, which are large soft-tissue masses that develop in pressure points. These nodules can be painful to walk on if they form on the weight-bearing surface of the foot, but they are benign, noncancerous masses. Rheumatoid can also affect the ankle joint in severe cases, causing similar symptoms of increased swelling, warmth, pain with rest, and movement.

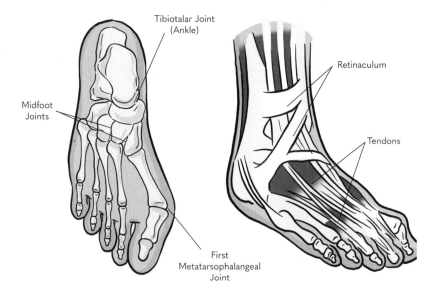

Rheumatoid factor is a blood test that is used in conjunction with other inflammatory lab markers to assist in the diagnosis of RA; however, lab work alone is not sufficient to diagnose RA. Criteria from a clinical, laboratory, and imaging standpoint must be met, according to the American College of Rheumatology, for you to be properly diagnosed with RA.

Like many other arthritides and autoimmune diseases, early diagnosis is important to delay progression of the disease. Starting patients on anti-inflammatories or disease-modifying medications can help control pain and discomfort. Intra-articular cortisone injections can be helpful in controlling joint flare-ups that are unresolved with oral medications. Offloading padding for rheumatoid nodules, if present, can help alleviate some pain and pressure. For severe cases where significant deformity is present, customized accommodative orthotics are beneficial to alleviate symptoms and prevent further problems.

Surgical procedures to treat rheumatoid arthritis aim to provide stability and improved function of the foot. Keeping patients ambulatory and able to perform the activities of daily living are the priorities. To address pain or severe arthritis of the big toe joint or the lesser toes, surgical options include a fusion of the joint, an implant to replace the joint, or an arthroplasty. A fusion removes the affected joint cartilage surfaces, allowing bone to fuse in the newly corrected position. This is a tried-and-true procedure for patients with RA, because a fusion does not allow for the recurrence of deformity when it heals. An arthrodesis (fusion) takes approximately six to eight weeks, partial to non-weight-bearing in a boot, to heal. An implant (total or semi joint replacement) involves placing a synthetic silicone joint in the affected joint to regain range of motion. Recovery typically is two to four weeks, partial weight bearing in a surgical shoe. This procedure is used cautiously in RA patients because their bodies can react adversely to the implant, causing more inflammation, pain, and poor incision healing. An arthroplasty involves removing the base of the proximal phalanx without the use of an implant, while additionally lengthening the extensor tendon, in most cases, to allow surgical offloading of the joint. Recovery for this procedure varies from two to six weeks, depending on whether a temporary wire is placed to hold the toe's position while it's healing. Keep in mind that having RA with or without medical management can slow the recovery process for any of these procedures, causing postoperative recovery time frames to vary.

If the rheumatoid nodules are painful, excising them can alleviate pain and improve mobility; recurrence, however, is always a possibility and should be discussed with the patient prior to surgery. The pan metatarsal head resection is the final procedure option for patients with severe rheumatoid arthritis deformity of the foot. This procedure is usually performed in conjunction with a fusion of the big toe joint. A pan metatarsal head resection removes the head of the lesser metatarsals, which in turn allows the toes to straighten while alleviating the pressure of the joint deformity. The toes can temporarily be pinned to prevent drifting postoperatively; however, temporary fixation is patient and surgeon dependent. The recovery for a pan metatarsal head resection is usually four to six weeks.

Possible complications with any surgery on a rheumatoid patient include infection, swelling, delayed healing, and pain. The possibility for recurrence of the deformity or pain is always something to be discussed with a patient suffering from RA. Although there are many surgical options available for RA patients, these procedures are only performed if there is pain associated with the affected joint that is unrelieved with conservative treatment, or if there is a direct effect on the patient's quality of life.

Osteoarthritis

Degenerative joint disease (DJD), "wear and tear" arthritis, and posttraumatic arthritis are all synonymous with osteoarthritis (OA). This type of arthritis can lead to pain, stiffness, and loss of motion in any joint it affects. While conservative measures typically treat the symptoms of OA and do not provide a "cure," it is still recommended to try conservative treatments prior to surgery.

OA develops due to overuse or an injury to any joint. The affected joint becomes swollen and painful. Decreased motion and pain are also associated with the joint as the disease progresses. Some patients describe a "grinding" or "crunching" sensation when they move the joint. Bone spurs, also called osteophytes, can develop around the joint as a reaction to chronic inflammation. The bone spur causes an abrupt end-range of motion to the joint, almost like the joint locks up and cannot move any further. Some joints, if left untreated, can become so severely arthritic that the cartilage surface of the joint is completely worn down and the body attempts to fuse itself. Osteoarthritis can also cause referred pain to other joints, because the loss of motion in one joint can cause other surrounding joints to pick up the motion lost, leading to pain.

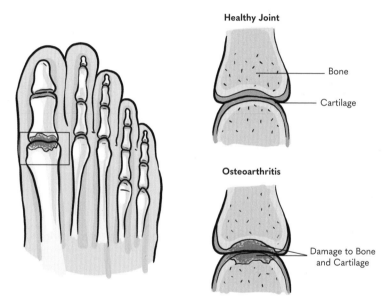

Healthy Joint

Bone

Cartilage

Osteoarthritis

Damage to Bone and Cartilage

Diagnosis of OA is both clinical and radiological. Evaluating an osteoarthritic joint in the office setting is fairly straightforward. Radiographically, joint space narrowing, flattening of the bones, and osteophytes are apparent. No blood tests or further imaging are typically required to verify an OA diagnosis.

Conservative treatments are targeted to decrease the pain and eliminate or control the motion of the joint. Keep in mind that the only way to get rid of the arthritis is surgery. There is no definitive treatment option to regrow cartilage in an arthritic joint. Biologic injections are undergoing research for the regeneration of cartilage; however, the research is still ongoing. Initially, oral anti-inflammatories or topical anti-inflammatories can be helpful, depending on the severity of the arthritis to the joint. Intra-articular cortisone injections are also available for episodes of acute flare-ups and may delay the need for surgical intervention. Viscosupplementation injections are a regenerative medicine option, used primarily in the knee and ankle joint, which have also delayed the need for surgery. The purpose of these injections is to provide lubrication to the joint, improving the range of motion as well as providing possible regenerative tissue effects. Other regenerative medicine options, such as platelet-rich plasma (PRP), can help reduce the pain in the affected joint as well, by stimulating new tissue growth and initiating the healing cascade of events. Finally, a custom orthotic can be beneficial for controlling and restricting motion in the affected joint, therefore eliminating the pain.

If conservative treatments fail, surgical intervention is usually warranted. If you have mild arthritic pain secondary to a bone spur, performing an exostectomy can be helpful. This procedure can be performed on almost any joint in the foot. It involves shaving down the prominent spurs to make them flat with the surrounding bone. The recovery is usually quick and easy, with partial weight bearing in a surgical shoe. The downside to this procedure is that it may only provide temporary relief; the bone spur can regrow since the arthritic joint itself was not surgically treated. If the joint is past the point of a bone spur shaving because it is too severely affected by arthritis, then two commonly performed procedures are available: an arthrodesis (joint fusion) or an arthroplasty with or without an implant (joint replacement). Both of these options can apply to most, but not all, joints in the foot and ankle.

An arthrodesis, commonly known as a joint fusion, is the first option to discuss with a podiatrist. The procedure entails removing the cartilaginous surface of the arthritic joint, aligning the two bones together, and forcing them to fuse with a combination of screws, plates, and pins. This procedure removes the joint motion altogether and prevents recurrence of arthritis to the joint in the long term, assuming no complications occur. A fusion is a more effective treatment for a younger patient population because it is a long-term fix with relatively high patient satisfaction for years after the procedure is healed. The recovery for a fusion is approximately six to eight weeks, usually non-weight-bearing in an immobilization boot or cast. A fusion is commonly performed in arthritic big toe joints, the midfoot, the heel, and the ankle for end-stage OA. Complications associated with this procedure include infection, swelling, nonunion (fusion does not heal), or malunion (fusion heals in a misaligned position).

An arthroplasty with joint replacement is the other option for OA of the foot or ankle. This procedure maintains motion at the joint and usually allows for a quicker recovery. A joint replacement recovery is usually two weeks for the small toes and six to eight weeks for the ankle. Joint replacements are reserved for older individuals because the shelf life is fluid, based on the activity of the individual. This is a conversation that should happen during a surgical consultation. An implant placed in a younger person has more potential to wear down faster and possibly cause more pain. In contrast, a joint replacement in an individual older than 60 will more likely outlast the patient and tolerate the age-related activity level. If you are younger and prefer to maintain motion in your joint with a joint replacement, keep in mind that a subsequent surgery will probably be needed in the future. This should be extensively discussed with your doctor, as an implant in the wrong type of patient can have detrimental complications. These complications include swelling, infection, and implant failure, which would then lead to a fusion or even possibly an amputation.

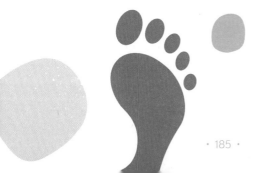

FAQs

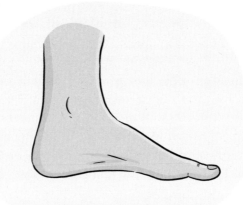

How do I know what kind of arthritis I have?

During a visit with your doctor, there are many ways to determine which type of arthritis you have. Utilizing blood work, imaging, family history, and a clinical exam are all important for determining the appropriate diagnosis.

I don't have pain. Do I need to do anything to help my arthritis?

Not really. If you don't have pain, you are lucky. I would recommend preventative measures, such as wearing a custom orthotic to prevent further breakdown and pain.

Do cortisone injections work for arthritis?

Yes. While a cortisone injection won't get rid of arthritis, it may make it feel better and prevent the need for more invasive treatments.

Should I see any other specialists if I have arthritis?

Yes. A team approach is important in helping to control your arthritic pains. Seeing a rheumatologist and your primary care doctor, in conjunction with a podiatrist, is a great way to manage your disease process.

Should I get a fusion or an implant?

This really comes down to your feelings on motion or no motion, and if you are willing to have potential secondary procedures performed as you get older. If you adamantly refuse to fuse a joint, then an arthroplasty with a joint implant is your only option. Implants can be successful in the right patient; however, secondary procedures may be indicated later on if the implant wears down or fails. If you are reluctant to have secondary procedures performed as you get older and want a "one and done" procedure, then a fusion is the better option.

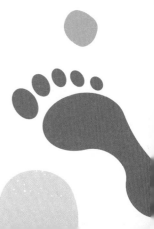

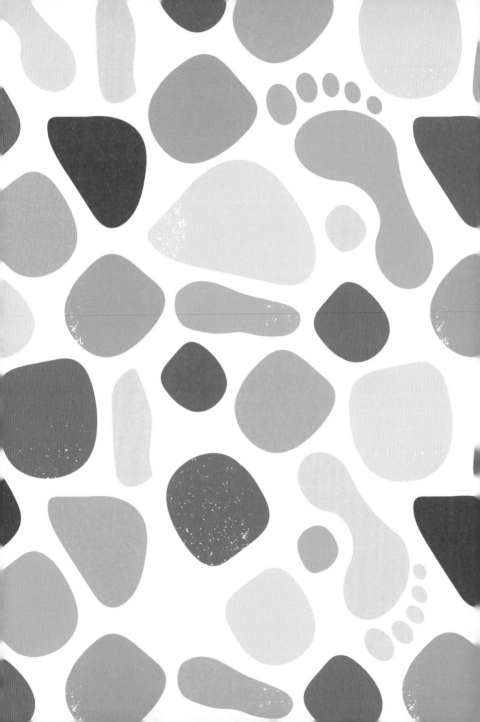

CHAPTER 17

PEDIATRIC FOOT PAIN

Four of the most common conditions encountered when treating kids' feet are ingrown nails, warts, toe walking, and heel pain. Ingrown toenails and warts have previously been discussed (see Chapters 7 and 10, respectively); therefore, this chapter will focus on toe walking and heel pain.

Toe Walking

Toe walking is one of the most common concerns parents seem to have when their children start walking. While toe walking is a finding in some neurological and musculoskeletal disorders, the majority of the time, toe walking is common practice among children learning to walk.

Toddlers just learning to walk at approximately 10 to 12 months of age commonly begin the process by walking more on their toes. This can occur well into toddlerhood, up to 3 years old. It is not necessarily an indicator that something is wrong. Toe walking can be a natural progression of developing a mature gait (walking). If your child is walking normally and suddenly starts toe walking at an older age, such as 10 years old or older, then he or she should be taken to a physician immediately for evaluation, as this can be an early sign of a neurological disorder. It is certainly advisable to have your child see a podiatrist to have it checked to help ease your mind, but rest assured that most of the time it is a normal finding.

During the initial evaluation for a toe walker, X-rays will usually be taken to eliminate a bone-related etiology. After X-rays are completed, a full gait evaluation will be performed, both while the child is standing and walking. If the child is able to rest the foot in a position where the heel touches the ground, then toe walking is flexible and should eventually resolve as the child's gait continues to become more like that of an adult. If the heel cannot touch the ground on manipulation of the foot, then further examination should be performed. A thorough range-of-motion exam of the ankle joint is usually performed, with both the knee extended and flexed, to determine if a certain muscle group is tight (equinus), causing the toe walking.

If the toe walking is due to a neurological or musculoskeletal problem, a neurology specialist is usually consulted for further evaluation. A neurologist may perform lab work or utilize specialized neurological tests in the office to determine whether the toe walking is secondary to cerebral palsy, muscular dystrophy, or a spinal cord abnormality. Conservative treatment, regardless of whether the toe walking is neurological or not, typically starts with bracing, stretching exercises, and physical therapy. Bracing improves the range of motion of the ankle joint and decreases the tightness of the Achilles, allowing for better heel contact during walking. Physical therapy would also be very worthwhile for gait training and range-of-motion exercises. If conservative treatment fails to resolve the toe walking, and it is from a known etiology such as equinus or a neurological disorder, then surgery is typically warranted. Surgery is aimed at lengthening the Achilles tendon to improve the range of motion at the ankle joint, allowing for proper heel strike and toe off during gait.

As stated earlier, the majority of kids that we treat for toe walking have no underlying condition. The main thing we stress to parents is to be patient, and to understand that the child will grow out of it as maturation of the gait occurs. How long? There is no definitive time frame. As long as the above-mentioned medical conditions have been ruled out, patience and persistence are key with toe walkers.

Pediatric Heel Pain

The most common podiatric problem we treat in children is heel pain. The term associated with heel pain in children is calcaneal apophysitis, also called growing pains or Sever's disease. Have no fear; it is not really a disease. It is simply inflammation of the growth plate on the heel.

The most common complaint with calcaneal apophysitis is "my child is in a lot of pain after sports." Other complaints include a child 's reluctance to participate in activities, or the presentation of limping with normal walking. Calcaneal apophysitis occurs in kids up to the point of skeletal maturity. For girls, the age range is usually around 13 to 15, while boys typically develop it around 14 to 16 years of age. Obviously, this can fluctuate from child to child. The pain is usually on the inside of the heel or the back of the heel, or with compression of the heel. The exact mechanics of calcaneal apophysitis are actually pretty simple. The Achilles tendon inserts on the top part of the growth plate, and the plantar fascia inserts on the bottom part of it. When your child is playing sports, a shearing force occurs across the growth plate due to the back-and-forth pull of the Achilles and plantar fascia. This action, coupled with pronation of the foot while walking, causes abnormal pulling, leading to inflammation of the growth plate on the heel.

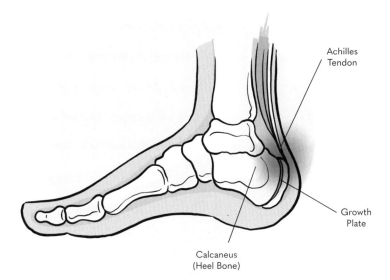

Achilles Tendon

Growth Plate

Calcaneus (Heel Bone)

The treatment of calcaneal apophysitis is never surgical. In fact, kids respond extremely well to conservative treatment. Basic RICE therapy, such as rest, anti-inflammatories, stretching, and icing, are great treatments to initiate. Stretching is essential for improvement. A runner's stretch and rolling the foot on a frozen water bottle for fifteen minutes is helpful. It can be difficult to get your child to perform these stretching activities, but if they are included in his or her normal routine, most kids will adapt to the changes. Just like everything else in podiatry, making sure the child has custom orthotics in their shoes and cleats will go a long way. Custom orthotics can rapidly improve the symptoms of calcaneal apophysitis, especially for kids in sports activities, as they provide better support to the plantar fascia and Achilles tendon. For severe cases of calcaneal apophysitis, abstinence from the sport may be needed, with immobilization in a boot or cast for two to four weeks.

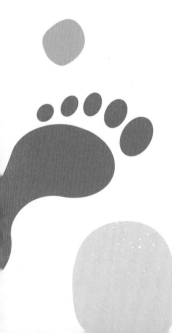

FAQs

I believe my child has growing pains. Should I just wait it out?

No, because these growing pains could continue until skeletal maturity. Stretching and icing are good to initiate; however, if the pain persists for more than seven to ten days, your child may need a good pair of custom orthotics.

Does my child need to continue with the orthotics if the pain goes away?

Yes. Even once they get to skeletal maturity, your child's foot type may be the cause for pain in the first place.

Should I get heavier shoes for my toe-walking child?

Have your child assessed first by a podiatrist. More likely than not, he or she won't need any shoe modifications. Most children outgrow toe walking as their gait becomes more normal.

How do I know if toe walking is something serious enough to be concerned about?

If your child can stand flat footed when he or she is not walking, then typically toe walking will slowly resolve as the child's gait matures.

Will surgery be needed to fix my child's heel pain?

No. Children rarely require surgical intervention for heel pain. Calcaneal apophysitis, the most common cause for heel pain in kids, can be fixed conservatively.

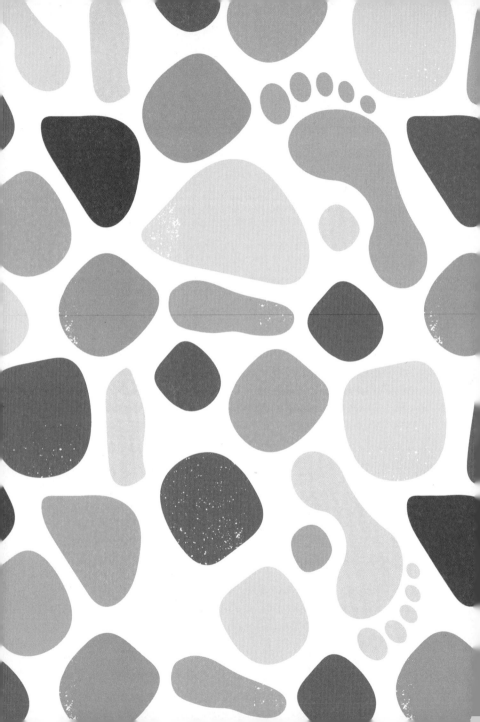

CHAPTER 18

DIABETES AND HOW IT AFFECTS FEET

In certain regions all over the world, complications associated with diabetes are often found in the top-ten causes of death. For those with diabetes, having a trusted podiatrist to help manage their symptoms and check their feet regularly is a must.

Diabetes is a multisystem disease process that is correlated to the glucose (sugar) in your body. If you are diabetic with uncontrolled glucose that runs high for an extended period of time, it can have a catastrophic effect on your body from head to toe. Managing diabetes requires a multidisciplinary medical approach, meaning that your diabetes will be treated by multiple specialists, as well as your primary care doctor. Maintaining your diabetes with diet and medication is very important. Because diabetes is such a huge topic to cover, I'm going to break it down based on systems and how it affects feet.

Vascular

In our feet, we have macrocirculation and microcirculation. The macrocirculation is the big blood vessels in the legs and feet, while the microcirculation is the smaller vessels in your toes. The first exam podiatrists perform on a diabetic patient involves checking for foot pulses. There is an artery on top of your foot and an artery behind the inside of your ankle. If your doctor can feel your pulses, then your macrocirculation is considered normal; however, just because these pulses are palpable does not necessarily mean that no vascular disease is present. You can have sufficient macrocirculation, but it does not tell us about your microcirculation, which can become compromised in patients with diabetes. Microcirculation is difficult to assess, but the clinical exam can help your doctor determine whether or not there is a concern present. Capillary fill time is a clinical exam that involves pinching the tip of the toe to see how long it takes to pink up. If your toe is slow to return back to a normal color (fewer than three seconds), then this could indicate microvascular disease. Another telltale sign of good versus bad circulation is the quality of your skin, nails, and hair growth. Do you lack hair halfway down your legs or on your toes? Is your skin tight and shiny in appearance? These may all be signs of poor circulation.

Patients who complain of pain in their toes may have poor blood flow. If small vessels in the toes are not getting oxygenated blood to the tissues, then the tissues start to become ischemic (painful) and risk necrosis (dead tissue). Typically, pain medication will help very little with vascular ischemia pain. The only way to improve the pain is to bring the blood supply back to the tissue as quickly as possible. This is performed via revascularization by a vascular surgeon. Other patient complaints include calf pain and pain when they lie in bed at night, with relief only achieved when they put their legs in a dependent (downward) position. The most severe symptom of ischemic pain is necrosis or gangrene of the tissue or toes. The skin turns a dark-red, dusky color initially, and then starts to turn black as tissue dies from a lack of oxygen in the blood. This is typically associated with end-stage vascular disease, which requires intervention, usually in the form of amputation.

So, what does diabetes have to do with this? Hyperglycemia (excess glucose levels) can inhibit the cells that induce dilation of the blood vessels, and it can also cause increased clotting signals, causing plaque to accumulate. Plaque can build up in your vessels, decreasing the flow of oxygenated blood to the tissue and leading to claudication (pain with walking) and further vascular disease. This is an important reason for establishing what a diabetic patient's circulation is like in his or her feet. If a small wound develops, the lack of circulation could lead to slower healing, increasing the risk of infection and amputation.

After a podiatrist does a thorough vascular exam, X-rays of the feet are usually taken for baseline imaging. Even though arteries and veins are soft tissue, calcification within the arterial walls can be dense enough to show on an X-ray. This is an indication of vascular disease, and a referral to a vascular surgeon should be done, regardless of whether good pulses are noted in the foot. Some tests, such as an ABI (ankle-brachial index), can give a good indication of the circulation in your lower extremities, from the thigh down to your big toe. An arteriogram can also be performed to show the vascular map of vessels winding down the legs. It can also identify areas in the arteries where runoffs are narrowed or completely blocked. If indicated, a vascular surgeon can perform an endovascular procedure to attempt opening up the vessels, removing any thickened plaques, or placing a stent in the vessel to keep it open to improve blood flow to the leg.

On the other end of the spectrum, your venous flow delivers blood back to the heart. This part of the vascular system can also become compromised by diabetes. Hyperglycemia can inhibit tissue in the veins from functioning properly, causing the valves within your veins to not work effectively. The veins, in turn, will not pump the blood back up like they should, causing more swelling to your feet and ankles. Gravity is not your friend in this situation because blood begins to pool in the legs when they are placed in a dependent position. This increased swelling associated with poor vein function can lead to ulcerations and "weeping," or drainage, from the skin. Therapeutic compression stockings are essential to control lower extremity swelling associated with venous insufficiency. Discuss getting a prescription for a pair with your doctor if you start to see signs of increased swelling or varicose veins in your feet and ankles.

The most important things you can do to prevent arterial disease is to control your blood sugar level and not smoke. If you smoke or use tobacco products, quitting can immediately improve oxygenation to the tissue. Diabetic patients who smoke can become riddled with vascular complications and risk amputation. Period. If you prevent the risk of plaque buildup, you prevent problems. Regular bimonthly monitoring by your podiatrist and an annual exam by a vascular doctor are essential for prevention. Prevention of what? In diabetics, it's preventing the amputation of a toe, your foot, or your leg.

Neurologic

As with the vascular network, there are large and small nerve fibers in your feet. The neurological system may be the most important and complex one when it comes to evaluating diabetics. When the glucose level in diabetics becomes elevated, it can cause a breakdown of the nerve fibers, resulting in neuropathy to the feet. The nerves in our body have an outer layer of myelin, which is, in essence, an insulator to protect the nerve. As the myelin starts to break down, it leads to a plethora of sensations that can occur with neuropathy. Other than what the patient tells us subjectively, podiatrists check for three specific nerve pathways: vibratory sensation, protective sensation, and proprioception.

To test vibratory sensation, a tuning fork is placed on a toe, from which a patient should feel a vibration. If the vibratory feeling is absent or is gone quickly, then you likely have neuropathy. Protective sensation involves using a small, fishing-line type of material to poke specific sites on the bottom of both feet. If you don't feel a certain amount of these sites, then you have neuropathy. Finally, proprioception is tested. A podiatrist will have you close your eyes and lift your big toe up or down. If you cannot identify which way your toe is lifted or you lack spatial awareness of where your toe is pointing, then this is a positive sign for neuropathy. With that said, you could pass all of these with flying colors and still have neuropathy symptoms. These tests are used for screening purposes only. They're a guideline. You could still have neuropathy, but it may be earlier in the disease stage, where testing does not pick up on it as well.

Presenting symptoms of patients with neuropathy is where things get interesting. The sensations a diabetic can feel with neuropathy are all over the place. To name a few, it can feel like sharp, shooting, burning, tingling, or numbing pain. Some describe it as "I'm stepping on sandpaper," or "it feels like there are ants in my feet," or even "it feels like a sock is bunched up in my foot." All of these descriptions, and many more, are very important to share with your podiatrist because they help home in on the diagnosis of neuropathy.

The signs and symptoms above are great ways to determine if someone has neuropathy. If indicated, other studies or tests can be performed to check for neuropathy, such as an electromyography test (EMG) or a biopsy of the superficial skin to check micro nerve fibers. Again, these tests can be helpful, but ultimately, neuropathy is a clinical diagnosis.

So what can neuropathy lead to? For starters, the primary problem with neuropathy is the unrelenting pain it brings to your feet. All of the symptoms mentioned above can make walking and getting around unbearable. Most people with neuropathy have worse pain at night before going to bed. If your neuropathy has caused numbness in your feet, it can be extremely hazardous. It is highly recommended to not walk barefoot if you have diabetes with neuropathy. If you step on something, whether it be a nail, a splinter, or hot pavement, it could lead to an abscess or ulceration, which precipitates further problems. The last condition caused by neuropathy is Charcot foot. Charcot, also known as neuropathic arthropathy, is the fragmentation or microfracturing of the bones in your foot. This breakdown, or microfracture, is believed to be due to the combination of good circulation and lack of feeling in the foot, causing the bones in your arch to fracture and, eventually, consolidate into a solid bony block. People with Charcot tend to present with a red, warm, swollen foot. Pain can present as well but is not always noted. Most Charcot patients develop the textbook appearance of a rocker bottom foot, where the bottom of the foot is convex. This is an issue because you are now walking on a prominent bone with no feeling, increasing the risk of ulceration, infection, or amputation.

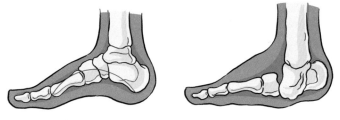

Normal Foot   Charcot Foot

If you develop Charcot, there are several treatment options available. If you are diagnosed with new-onset Charcot (acute Charcot), then immobilization in a CROW (Charcot restraint orthotic walker) boot is imperative. This device is customized to your foot type, to ensure a proper fit and to alleviate abnormal pressure to the foot while it is healing. Serial X-rays are performed to monitor the progression of the Charcot, ensuring that healing is seen. Typically, you see bone breakdown initially, followed by the start of bone healing and then coalescence (consolidation of bone). Once X-rays show good coalescence of bone, and clinically acute symptoms have resolved, then you can be transferred to shoes with custom accommodative orthotics. This is important; because of the convex nature of the bottom of the foot, you may be more prone to ulcers forming. You can get flare-ups of acute Charcot, after everything appears well healed, to the same foot or the other foot, which is why diabetics with Charcot need to see a podiatrist on a regular basis. Surgery to realign the foot into a more normal position is also a treatment option; however, there is controversy as to whether surgery truly helps when bone quality is poor to begin with and may not heal well. Further breakdown is common, and complications can be high. Amputation is not uncommon for a patient with Charcot because of the progressive nature of the disease.

Prevention is the best way to avoid neuropathy, by maintaining your blood glucose levels early on in your diagnosis of diabetes. Once you get neuropathy, there is no undoing it. Treating neuropathy is based on your symptoms and the severity of them. Topical and oral medications are available to improve neuropathy pain, but they will not cure it. The medications are meant to help stop the aforementioned symptoms to make it easier for you to walk around or sleep at night. Medications provide improvement for some patients but can be ineffective for others. Working with your podiatrist and primary care doctor is important for evaluating which medication, if any, is right for you.

Control your blood sugars, avoid going barefoot, and monitor your feet daily. Neuropathy can be a turbulent complication associated with diabetes and shouldn't be overlooked by you or your doctor.

Musculoskeletal

The musculoskeletal system evaluates deformities that pertain to the feet with regard to range of motion of the joints and muscle strength. Charcot foot, as previously discussed, can cause major deformity of the feet, increasing your risk for wounds and a nonfunctional foot; however, Charcot is not the only deformity secondary to diabetic neuropathy. Diabetic neuropathy can cause nerves that control your foot muscles to stop functioning, as well leading to other deformities such as hammertoes, bunions, and flatfeet.

The most concerning reason to evaluate these deformities that are secondarily caused by diabetes is that the deformities become a focal point of pressure. If a diabetic, neuropathic patient develops increased pressure, the skin can break down, which can then lead to ulcerations, infections, and amputations. Weakness of a muscle group over another muscle group can decrease range of motion and cause excess pressure on parts of the foot and ankle as well. Radiological evaluation coupled with the presence or absence of arthritic changes is key to determining the severity of these deformities.

Conservative care for foot deformities associated with the diabetic foot typically utilizes offloading padding or accommodative orthotics. A majority of insurance will cover diabetic shoes and custom orthotics, which are soft and help to alleviate pressure from those points. For digital contractures, such as hammertoes or bunions, offloading pads can be used to reduce pressure to these areas at high risk for ulceration.

If you have an amputation on your foot, custom orthotics can be made with fillers that fill the void left by the absent toes and/or foot. Surprisingly, the use of fillers and physical therapy can assist with very little change in your gait with an amputation. From the standpoint of amputations, the procedure will go as far back as the joint called the Chopart joint. If you require a more proximal amputation after this, it is usually a below-knee amputation. The main reason that an amputation isn't performed between these two levels is because the limb becomes nonfunctional. Having a below-the-knee amputation allows for getting a prosthetic if the patient is still capable of ambulation. Patients tend to be more functional with a prosthetic limb just below the knee than an amputation any farther back than the midfoot.

Although the musculoskeletal exam is less complicated than the vascular or neurological exams, it is still imperative to perform a full exam on every patient with diabetes. When appropriately identifying the problematic conditions noted above and discussing preventative treatment, it can improve a diabetic patient's quality of life and overall satisfaction of care.

Dermatologic

Last, but certainly not least, is the dermatologic evaluation. This includes a thorough skin and nail evaluation. When checking the skin, a doctor will look for any open sores, blisters, cuts, or ulcerations. A check for suspicious lesions is also done; even looking between the toes is important. Of course, a thorough exam of the nails is also helpful for treatment purposes.

Because diabetics have a poor immune system, checking for cuts, abrasions, and ulcerations is very important. It could be a blister from an ill-fitting shoe, a cut from dropping something on your foot, or a scrape from hitting your foot against something you may not even be aware of. Small cuts, scrapes, and abrasions can lead to bigger problems in patients with diabetes with neuropathy. All of the aforementioned scenarios, if left untreated, could lead to infections and therefore worsening wounds that become deeper. Poor wound healing secondary to diabetes, in addition to poor circulation or neuropathy, is a recipe for disaster. If wounds are not monitored closely to ensure appropriate healing is noted, they can become deeper, leading to infection of the bone (osteomyelitis). Bone infection is difficult to treat and requires intravenous antibiotics and, most times, an amputation of the affected toe or limb. It is important, as a diabetic, never to underestimate any small cut.

As podiatrists, we perform a full dermatologic exam from the knee down to the toenails. Checking between the toes is also very important. Between the toes, also called the webspace, is a common spot for moisture to collect; if too much moisture collects it can lead to ulcerations and infections. Between the toes is an area often forgotten by most people when checking the feet daily. Sometimes macerated (wet) webspaces can be very tender; however, diabetic neuropathy may mask this pain, and many patients will not even know a wound is present. Drying well between the toes is important after you shower to prevent breakdown.

Callus formation is the last skin condition that can occur on the feet, which can cause problems for a diabetic patient. Calluses form on pressure points. If the callus is not properly treated, the friction continues, leading to further breakdown of the skin. The callus blisters and separates from the underlying skin. As this happens over a period of time, the shearing of the callus/blister gets deeper, and then the formation of a larger, deeper ulceration can develop. As the ulcer gets deeper, the risk of infections and amputations elevates exponentially.

Toenail fungus is also commonly seen in diabetic patients, due to the suppression of their immune system. The increased thickness of the nail can cause more pressure on the toe, which can lead to more pain in the toes. The thickness and incurvation of the nail can lead to an ingrown nail as well. The thickness of the nail can cause rubbing on a shoe, and the shearing force can cause the nail to loosen or fall off.

It is imperative as a diabetic that you have your feet checked regularly, not just at home but by a podiatrist as well. Checking for new cuts, blisters, or abrasions is important. I always tell my diabetic patients that no problem is too small. I would rather they come to see me, and have it only turn out to be a minor problem, rather than ignoring it and progressing to a severe infection, or worse, an amputation. Most important, all insurance allows you to visit your podiatrist every nine weeks for a full diabetic evaluation and treatment if you have diabetes with a complication of neuropathy, vascular disease, or a history of amputation. Allow your podiatrist to shave your calluses or trim your nails on a regular basis to prevent you from cutting yourself, which could lead to infection or amputation. Because some diabetics have no feeling in their feet, they may not even know they cut themselves. This starts the vicious cycle of cut, infection, and amputation.

Diabetes is one of the most damaging diseases we see in our field. I can't stress enough how important it is to control your blood sugars and be checked by a podiatrist regularly. For diabetics, including a podiatrist within your multidisciplinary team of physicians is important. Other physicians you should consider consulting with if you are diabetic, even if it is for maintenance purposes, are an endocrinologist, ophthalmologist, vascular surgeon, neurologist, dietician, and even a psychologist.

FAQs

Why is it important to see a podiatrist as a diabetic?

If you start seeing a podiatrist early in the diagnosis of diabetes, the goal is the prevention of complications; having a full foot evaluation helps to determine if there are any problems with your circulation, nerves, muscle function, or skin.

Why do I get burning, tingling, or numbness to my toes?

You have neuropathy. Neuropathy occurs in patients with diabetes due to fluctuating or poorly controlled blood sugar. There is no fix for neuropathy, only treating the symptoms; therefore, it is imperative to responsibly manage your blood sugar so you don't develop this complication.

What if I have poor circulation? What can a podiatrist do for me?

Most likely, you won't know you have poor circulation until a foot exam is performed; therefore, having a podiatrist check your feet may be the first step toward finding out what your vascular road map looks like.

How often should I see my podiatrist?

Insurance allows diabetics with vascular disease, neuropathy, or a history of amputation to see a podiatrist every nine weeks; however, if there is ever something you are concerned about as a diabetic, you should be seen right away.

Does having diabetes mean that I will end up losing part of my foot?

No. If you exercise, watch what you eat, and take care of your blood sugars, you can live a completely normal, healthy life being a diabetic.

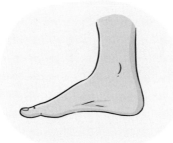

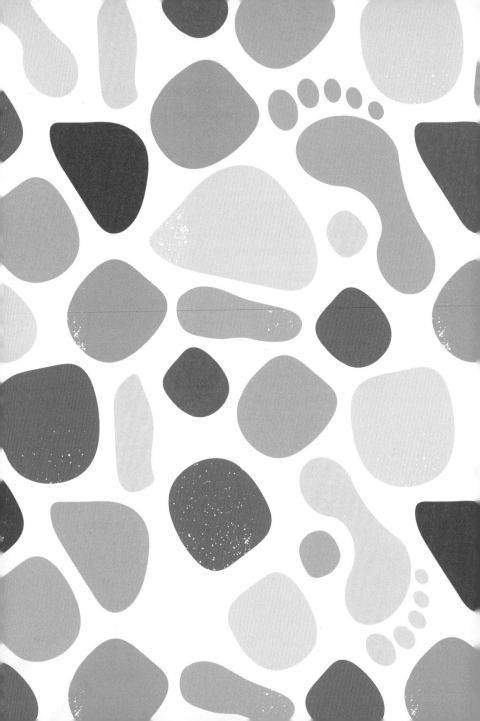

CHAPTER 19

SPORTS INJURIES AND TREATMENTS

While the list of potential foot and ankle sports-related injuries is long, this chapter covers the top five injuries seen in our office. For each injury, we will discuss the mechanism of injury, presentation, treatments, and prevention methods.

Subungual Hematoma

A subungual hematoma is a fancy term used to describe blood under the toenail. A hematoma can develop under the nail from direct trauma, or it can occur from the chronic use of blood thinners. A subungual hematoma is a common condition that can occur in most sporting activities.

The cause of a subungual hematoma is usually shoe gear related. Whether you are playing tennis or soccer, if your shoe or cleat is too tight, it will rub against your toe, causing friction to the nail plate. This friction causes the nail plate to detach from the underlying nail bed, allowing blood to collect underneath it. Subungual hematomas can also happen if the shoe or cleat is too big, causing a back-and-forth motion in the shoe. The constant microtrauma of motion and friction can lead to the subungual hematoma. Foot pathologies such as hammertoes and bunions may predispose you to developing a subungual hematoma, due to the deformity rubbing in shoes. Finally, a subungual hematoma can develop by direct trauma from someone stepping on your toe with a cleat. This instant trauma causes separation of the nail, followed by an accumulation of blood.

Upon initial presentation, the patient usually develops pain and drainage from the affected toe. Local redness may be noted around the nail plate itself, and the nail may feel soft. Occasionally, you can get tenting of the skin near the cuticle if the nail was impacted. The nail is usually a dark black color as the blood begins to clot. Odor is not commonly associated with a subungual hematoma.

The general rule of thumb states that if the subungual hematoma occupies more than 25 percent of the nail, the nail should be removed entirely to release pressure from the blood collecting under the nail. Yes, over time the nail will probably fall off on its own, but there are certain conditions that call for having the nail removed. First, if direct trauma occurred, then the nail should be removed to inspect for a cut or laceration under the nail that should be repaired. If your toe is stepped on, there is always a chance that a laceration could develop. Second, due to the dirty environment of the shoe and toenail, an infection can occur. If you allow the dried blood to sit under a relatively loose nail, you are at a higher risk of an infection. But do not drill a hole in your nail. If your nail falls off, do not allow anyone to suture it back in place. Yes, this has been done, and it defeats the purpose of removing the nail. The nail will grow back over time, and after taking a couple of weeks to heal, you won't even know anything happened.

So how do you prevent a hematoma from developing? Finding properly fitting shoes is imperative. You should have about a thumb's width of space between the end of your longest toe and the shoe. Notice I said the longest toe. If your second toe is longer than your first, fit your shoe to the second toe.

Unfortunately, there is no way to prevent someone from stepping on your toe; that is just a part of playing sports.

Turf Toe

Turf toe is a sprain of the metatarsophalangeal joint (MPJ) secondary to an injury sustained to the ligaments while playing sports. You may hear the term a lot while watching or playing sports, but what exactly is turf toe?

The injury occurs when the toe is hyperextended secondary to some type of direct impact. An example would be when a football player plants his toes down and heel off the ground; then he is tackled from behind, forcibly pushing the toe in an upward or dorsiflexed position. Wearing cleats makes players more susceptible to turf toe, due to the abrupt stop of the cleat on the playing field. Athletes commonly suffer a turf toe injury when playing soccer, football, rugby, and basketball. This injury can be devastating to a player. It should not be ignored, and it should be treated similarly to any other musculoskeletal injury.

The initial presentation of turf toe is usually accompanied by pain, swelling, and lack of motion. The big toe is usually the affected joint, as it receives the most impact of force when the foot is planted to the ground. The pain is centered primarily around the first metatarsophalangeal joint, aka the big toe joint. The pain is circumferential, meaning the entire joint usually hurts. The motion to the joint is typically guarded, with the player apprehensive to move it. A noticeable limp is

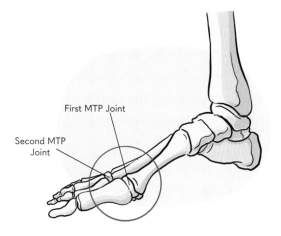

First MTP Joint

Second MTP
Joint

present as well, because propulsion through the big toe joint
is absent due to the pain. Certain motions, like changing di-
rection or pivoting, may be tough to perform because of the
pain elicited in the joint.

Treatment for turf toe is limited, and early diagnosis is key
in preventing long-term problems. For mild turf toe injuries,
taping the toe to prevent dorsiflexion may be helpful. Wearing
proper orthotics and/or stiff-soled shoes to eliminate motion
is also helpful. As with any other injury, anti-inflammatories
and icing are beneficial. If the injury is more severe, physical
therapy may be required to reduce the inflammation and improve the range of motion. Immobilization in a walking boot
may also be helpful in the more severe cases, specifically with
professional athletes who rely heavily on their propulsion,
often cutting and pivoting with their feet. If left untreated,

long-term complications could lead to arthritic changes to the joint. Turf toe recovery could range from a couple of weeks to a couple of months, depending on the severity of the injury.

While there is no way to prevent someone from falling on your foot while playing sports, having shoes with a rigid sole helps to reduce the risk of hyperextension to the joint. Orthotics in a shoe or cleat are helpful for everyday foot health, allowing the foot to function in a more efficient manner.

Sprained Ankle

Probably the most common sports injury we see in the office is an ankle sprain. An ankle sprain can be a debilitating injury that keeps you off the field or court if it is not addressed in a timely manner.

Ankle sprains occur when your ankle rolls inward or outward abruptly, stressing the ligaments around the ankle joint. A sprain can occur on the basketball court while jumping for a ball and coming down on your foot wrong, or it can occur when playing sports on uneven surfaces. Whether it is stepping in a hole or on a small hill, your foot rolls in while your ankle stays put, placing extra stress on the three major ligaments that comprise the outer part of your ankle joint. These three major ligaments on the outside of your ankle act as stabilizers for walking and running, keeping your ankle and foot in the proper position. Excess force of your body weight rolling over it causes these easily injured ligaments to give way. There are three grades to an ankle sprain: one, two, and three. These correspond to the number of ligaments that are injured. A grade one ankle sprain only involves the first ligament, and so on. The higher the grade, the more severe the sprain.

The initial presentation varies, depending on the severity of the ankle sprain. For mild ankle sprains, a limp may not even be present, whereas more severe sprains may inhibit the patient from putting pressure on the foot. Following the initial injury, the ankle will become extremely swollen. Some patients describe the swelling "like the size of a softball," followed by bruising that can extend from your ankle down your foot. Pain with range of motion of the ankle is easily

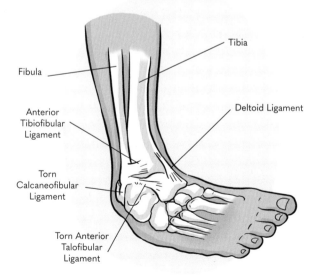

Fibula

Tibia

Anterior
Tibiofibular
Ligament

Deltoid Ligament

Torn
Calcaneofibular
Ligament

Torn Anterior
Talofibular
Ligament

found with most patients and can make it difficult to perform an assessment of each ligament. Attempting to palpate the ligaments can cause pain and tenderness as well. With an acute ankle sprain, a more detailed examination of the ankle ligaments and ankle joint range of motion may be delayed until the swelling and pain are improved after the initial injury.

Once you injure or sprain your ankle, you are at a much higher risk of doing it again because the ligaments become more lax and attenuated (stretched out). This inhibits the proprioceptive cells in the ligaments, making balance on the ankle more difficult. This new onset of laxity to the ligaments can result in long-term instability to the ankle.

For acute injuries that are mild in nature, follow the RICE treatment method: rest, ice, compression, and elevation. Decreasing the swelling will help with the pain and mobility. Using an elastic bandage wrap or ankle brace is also helpful for stability purposes and healing following the initial injury. For more severe injuries, immobilization in a walking boot may be necessary to allow the area to heal and to prevent excess motion and continued pain. Although X-rays are of minimal help with acute injuries, they are important to rule out any type of fracture. Detailed imaging of the ligaments is performed with an MRI. Sometimes patients with suspected instability can be taken to an imaging center for stress testing of the joint; however, this can be uncomfortable for the patient and may require sedation.

For chronic ankle instability following an ankle sprain, or for the athlete that suffers an acute rupture of the ligaments, surgery may be necessary for faster healing and better stability. Lateral ankle stabilizations are a category of procedures designed to repair the torn ligaments. These procedures utilize several methodologies. The most common procedures include primary repair with or without the use of augmented tape to reinforce the repair, and a repair with the utilization of a cadaveric or harvested tendon graft. Depending on the severity of the injury and the type of repair performed, recovery can vary from four to six weeks in a walking boot with physical therapy.

The best way to prevent ankle sprains is by either taping your ankle or using an ankle brace. As we discussed above, if you injure your ankle, you will be more susceptible to doing it again because of the instability or laxity to the ankle. Knowing this, you should always consider wearing an ankle brace or splint when participating in sports.

Achilles Rupture

Probably the most feared of all sports injuries is the Achilles rupture. A devastating injury followed by a long recovery could certainly change the scope of your long-term athletic plans.

An Achilles rupture occurs when you plant your foot and push off to jump or propel forward. This sudden, quick motion causes increased strain to the Achilles, which can result in a rupture. The rupture most commonly occurs at what's known as the watershed area, the portion of the Achilles with the least vascular supply. It usually occurs about four to six centimeters above the insertion point on your heel bone and is commonly known as the heel cord.

Upon initial presentation, pain and swelling usually encompass the entire back side of the leg, making it difficult to palpate the tendon. Bruising is typically observed around the rupture site. An Achilles rupture will hinder a patient's ability to point the toes down or push off with resistance on exam. A common test utilized is the "Homan's test," which involves squeezing the calf muscle without notable plantar flexion of the toes. Finally, a palpable dell is typically found; a doctor will run his or her finger along the Achilles tendon and feel a void at the rupture site. All of these findings are consistent with an Achilles rupture.

The main treatment for an Achilles rupture is to primarily repair it. If it is addressed as soon as possible after the initial injury, the two ends can usually be pulled back together in order to reapproximate them with sutures. If you wait too long, a graft may sometimes be required to fill the void between the two ruptured segments. The aftercare for an Achilles rupture is long and tiring. Expect to be off your foot for at least two to three months. Progressive weight bearing in a boot with the assistance of crutches follows soon after. Transition back to a shoe and physical therapy are usually the final stage of treatment. All in all, expect to be back to "normal" after ten to twelve months. Most patients experience a degree of weakness to the calf muscle after the injury, which is why physical therapy is initiated early in the postoperative healing process. However, just because you sustain a rupture does not mean you will not be active again. Older individuals who sustain an Achilles rupture, or individuals who are poor surgical candidates, usually are placed in a plantar flexed cast to allow the Achilles tendon to scar down and heal. Some studies suggest that casting and early physical therapy can be just as effective as surgery for this patient population.

Stretching and wearing proper orthotics are the best ways to prevent an Achilles rupture, especially in sports that place excessive strain on the Achilles tendon. Know your limits! If you don't feel physically fit or mobile enough to play a sport, don't push it. An Achilles rupture can be a disastrous condition that requires patience and determination to treat.

Toe Fracture

I'm pretty sure everyone reading this book has jammed their toe into a piece of furniture, issued a select choice of words, then immediately knew their toe was broken. Patients in this situation often tell us, "I don't need to go to a doctor. They won't do anything anyway."

The most common location for a toe fracture is the fifth toe, typically after catching it on a piece of furniture or another unmovable object. Dropping heavy objects on your toes is also a good way to end up with a fracture. Not all fractures are treated the same, which is why it is still worthwhile to visit a podiatrist if your toe does find the bed leg in the middle of the night.

Swelling, bruising, and pain are all very common findings with a toe fracture; depending on the severity of the fracture, toes will sometimes be pointing in different directions, known as dislocated/subluxed. Wearing shoes is difficult if not impossible following a toe fracture, and local numbness or tingling is also possible.

If you have a simple toe fracture, icing and buddy splinting to the nearest toe is usually the right answer. Wearing a stiff-soled, wide shoe is also helpful to alleviate pressure in the direct area. Complications of a broken toe requiring further medical attention include displacement, dislocation, or subluxation to the toe. Once verified both clinically and radiographically, the toe is anesthetized and reduced into proper position, followed by taping and a surgical shoe. The longer the break is present without medical intervention, the harder it is to reduce in-office. If you are unable to reduce a toe fracture because it has been a week or so since the injury, surgical intervention may be warranted to open the toe and reduce it properly to prevent posttraumatic arthritis. If the dislocation or fracture is severe, a screw and/or pin may be placed in the toe to hold it in the proper position.

How do you prevent a toe fracture? Maybe slippers with headlights?

Jones Fracture

The Jones fracture has become a more common fracture over the years, and more and more athletes seem to be suffering from it. Everyone hears about it, but does anyone know truly what a Jones fracture is?

Similar to an ankle sprain, the mechanism of injury is a forceful roll of the foot or ankle while playing sports on an unforgiving surface, e.g., a basketball court. As the foot rolls inward on the ankle, the soft tissue holds strong, forcing a fracture to occur near the base of the fifth metatarsal. Usually the biggest concern with this fracture is the location. The fracture occurs at an area of the fifth metatarsal with a poor blood supply, therefore leading to delayed healing and/or the need for surgical intervention, sometimes regardless of whether or not the fracture is displaced.

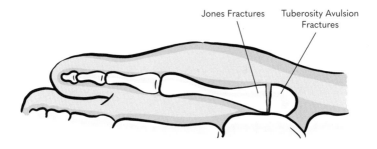

Jones Fractures · · · Tuberosity Avulsion Fractures

Pain is unavoidable near the outside of your foot. A heavy limp usually accompanies swelling, bruising, and a lack of motion. The verification of a Jones fracture is done by X-ray, CT scan, or both.

Treatment for a Jones fracture again depends on the age and activity level of the patient. For a professional athlete, a younger individual, or someone who is highly active, surgical repair is required. Luckily, it usually takes one screw to reapproximate the fracture site with a small incision. After about six to eight weeks in a boot, the fracture should be healed, and you can be transitioned back to regular shoes. For the older, more sedentary population, immobilization may be the treatment of choice, allowing the body to heal by secondary bone callus formation. If six to eight weeks go by with minimal progress noted, surgical intervention may be warranted at that time. If you are keen to avoid surgery and the site does not appear to be healing properly, a bone stimulator can be used to aid in the healing process. This device is placed on the outside of the foot, providing magnetic poles that align the bone cells to heal more uniformly. It can be a useful modality for any fracture with delayed healing, but it is especially useful for a Jones fracture.

The best way to prevent an injury like this is to wear proper support and/or orthotics in your shoes, as well as ankle support if you have a history of ankle sprains.

FAQs

If I have blood under my toenail, can I just poke a hole in the nail to drain it?

No. There are two reasons to avoid this method. One, the nail bed should be examined to assure that there is no laceration or open fracture under the nail. Two, removing an injured nail or loose nail after a hematoma will decrease the risk of an infection.

What are long-term complications of an ankle sprain or multiple ankle sprains?

Ankle instability is the biggest concern following an ankle sprain. Being proactive and wearing an ankle brace or taping your ankle is the best way to avoid further complications, such as the thickening of the ligaments or ankle joint arthritis.

Is there any way to avoid an Achilles tendon rupture?

While there is no specific way to guarantee you won't rupture your Achilles, stretching and wearing proper shoes and orthotics are the best ways to decrease the risk of rupture.

Nothing can be done for a toe fracture, correct?

Not necessarily. It depends on the severity of the fracture and what your X-rays look like. Clinically your toe may look fine, but an X-ray may reveal a displaced fracture that, if not treated, could lead to posttraumatic arthritis/stiffness of the toe.

I suffered a Jones fracture. Do I need surgery?

Unless it is a medical emergency, no one can force you into surgery. It is ultimately your decision. With that said, listen to what your physician recommends. Young, healthy patients will most likely want to have this fracture fixed to reduce the risk of chronic pain to a nonhealing fracture site.

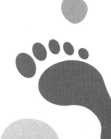

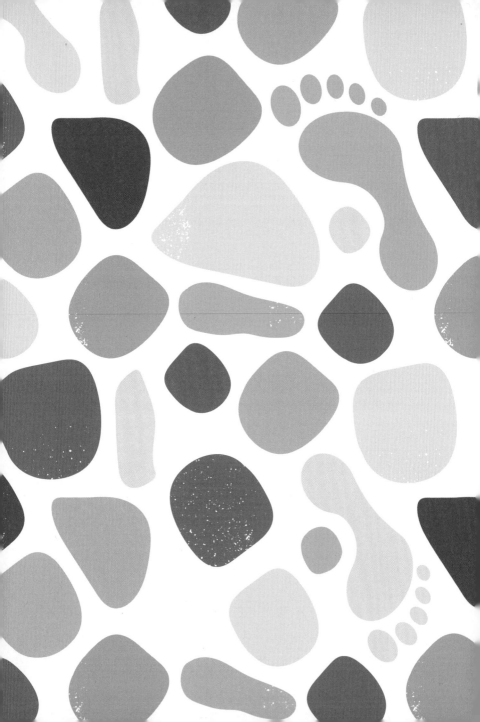

CHAPTER 20

SKIN CANCERS OF THE FOOT

Skin cancer can affect your entire body, but we will specifically discuss the three types of skin cancer encountered in the lower extremities, and how each is treated. Having a thorough skin exam by a podiatrist is imperative to check for any unforeseen suspicious skin lesions.

Basal Cell Carcinoma

Basal cell carcinoma (BCC) is the most common type of skin cancer found on the body. It develops from prolonged exposure to sun or tanning beds. Surprisingly, many people forget to put sunblock on their lower legs and feet when heading to the beach or pool, placing the lower extremities at risk for too much sun exposure. The initial presentation of basal cell cancer is commonly described as a pearly papule. It can present with small blood vessels running through it as well. These are obvious clinical exam findings that an experienced podiatrist will be looking for when performing a lower extremity skin exam.

While it is unlikely that basal cell carcinoma will become more invasive beyond the depth of the fat layer of the skin or result in death, it is still a condition that should be promptly addressed when found. Basal cell carcinoma is definitively diagnosed with a punch or shave biopsy in the office. The suspicious nevus (mole) is anesthetized, the biopsy is taken, and it is sent to a pathology lab to confirm the diagnosis. If you receive a positive result for basal cell carcinoma, then surgical excision is recommended. This can usually be performed under local anesthesia; however, if the lesion is large,

the patient can be taken to a surgery center for more comfort, using sedation with local anesthesia.

When surgical excision of a basal cell carcinoma is performed, a wide excision is done in order to ensure the
margins are clear of any cancerous cells. The area is usually
closed with a suture or sometimes left to heal in via secondary intention, i.e., like an open wound would heal.

Again, while the chances of cancer metastases or death from
basal cell carcinoma are extremely rare, it is still recommended to have the skin cancer excised when it is found. Those
with fair skin or prolonged exposure to the sun are at a much
higher rate of developing basal cell carcinoma, so using proper sunscreen while outside is always recommended.

Squamous Cell Carcinoma

Squamous cell carcinoma (SCC) is the second most common
type of skin cancer encountered in the field of podiatry. The
primary cause of SCC is sun exposure for prolonged periods
of time. SCC takes months to develop and usually appears as
a small cut or ulcer on the leg and/or foot. It is very common
for patients to complain that they have a small cut or spot on
their leg that keeps bleeding and won't heal. This is a telltale
sign for attention to be warranted for a biopsy. For patients
with ulcerations secondary to other conditions, such as diabetes or venous ulcers, there is a risk that the ulceration can
develop into a cancerous lesion; therefore, if a wound is not
responding to proper wound care, has enlarged or changed

significantly, or has become painful, then a biopsy of the ulcer is recommended. The longer you have an ulcer open on your foot, ankle, or leg, the higher risk you have of that ulcer becoming cancerous. Unlike basal cell carcinoma, if squamous cell carcinoma is left untreated it can progress, albeit slowly, and metastasize to different areas of your body.

A biopsy is used to confirm the diagnosis of squamous cell carcinoma. If you have a larger lesion or a nonhealing ulceration, sometimes multiple biopsies are taken to get a better idea as to whether there is concern for cancer. For larger ulcerations, it is not unusual for only a portion of the ulcer to have cancerous cells, which is why it is important to biopsy multiple spots in the ulcer.

As with basal cell carcinoma, surgical excision of a squamous cell carcinoma is performed once a biopsy has positively identified it. Usually, if the cancerous cells have not gone into the subcutaneous fat layer below the skin, then metastasis is unlikely to occur. If you have a lesion, mole, or wound that is not treated with excision, it could progress to a more invasive, dangerous cancer.

Melanoma

The least common, but most deadly, of the skin cancers encountered in the lower extremities is melanoma. The most important point to emphasize with melanoma is early detection. The earlier that melanoma is identified and removed, the better the prognosis. There are multiple types of melanoma, but for the purposes of this chapter, we will discuss the key characteristics every doctor uses to identify melanoma of the skin.

Melanoma is caused by ultraviolet light damage of the melanocytes, the pigment-producing cells in the skin. Melanoma can develop from a nevus (mole); therefore, consistent skin checks are important.

When determining whether a nevus on the lower leg is melanoma, a podiatrist takes into account the "**A, B, C, D, E**s" of the lesion. "**A**" stands for asymmetry. Is the lesion itself asymmetric? Is one side larger than the other, or is it shaped oddly? These are characteristics of a melanoma. "**B**" stands for border. Is the border of the lesion irregular, or does it have sharp corners to it? Melanoma exhibits these characteristics. "**C**" stands for color. If the lesion on your lower extremity is one solid color, it is unlikely to be a skin cancer; however, if it is multicolored, the risk of melanoma certainly increases. "**D**" stands for diameter. If the size of the lesion is larger than 6 mm, or the size of a pencil eraser, then melanoma should be considered. Finally, "**E**" stands for evolving. Has the lesion changed significantly over time? An example would be a tiny mole developing quickly into a black spot on your skin. If a significant change has occurred to the area, get it checked out.

A thorough inspection of your skin by a podiatrist is of vital importance because there is a melanoma that can develop under the nail plate: subungual melanoma. This type of melanoma is easily overlooked, as many doctors do not look closely at their patients' feet. If you develop a dark spot under your nail with no history of damage and color changes affecting the skin nearby, you should be seen by your podiatrist for concern of subungual melanoma. If your podiatrist is concerned as well, then the nail is removed to determine if the color changes are indeed to the nail bed (skin under the nail) or just the nail itself. If the color changes are only to the nail, there is no need to worry; however, if the nail bed has color changes as well, the suspicion for melanoma increases significantly. The musician Bob Marley died after developing a melanoma under his toenail. If left untreated, this type of melanoma can be aggressive and deadly.

A local biopsy is typically performed to determine if the lesion is truly melanoma or not. The biopsy will give you some insight on the depth of the melanoma, but further excision is required. If the biopsy comes back positive for melanoma, an oncology referral is immediately given to the patient for further evaluation. Additional imaging and a lymph node biopsy may be performed. If melanoma is on the tip of your toe or under your toenail, the treatment is usually amputation of the toe, as well as chemotherapy if lymph node involvement has already occurred. Losing your toe is a small price to pay when your life is at stake. Patients that have successfully undergone surgery to excise melanoma will be checked once to twice a year for the rest of their lives, to ensure that no other suspicious lesions develop again.

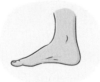

FAQs

I have an ulcer on my leg that is not healing. Should I be concerned?

Yes. If there is a spot that continues to bleed and not heal, there is high suspicion for squamous cell carcinoma of the skin.

Is the prognosis good with skin cancers in the lower extremities?

If caught early, yes. While melanoma progresses more rapidly, early detection with any cancer is helpful.

I'm concerned about a spot on my leg. What should I look for?

Remember the A, B, C, D, Es: Asymmetry, Border irregularity, Color variable, Diameter (more than 6 mm), and Evolving over time.

How do you confirm a cancerous diagnosis?

A biopsy is performed to definitively diagnose skin cancer.

I noticed a black spot on my toe. What should I do?

Get it checked immediately. Time is of the utmost urgency when it comes to melanoma diagnosis and treatment.

About the Authors

Dr. Todd Brennan and Dr. Leslie Johnston are a married podiatric couple practicing in Tampa, Florida. They met at The Ohio College of Podiatric Medicine, now known as Kent State University College of Podiatric Medicine.

Dr. Brennan owns Healthy Feet Podiatry, the most popular podiatric group on YouTube, with nearly 400,000 subscribers. He has also been voted the best podiatrist in Tampa multiple years in a row. Dr. Brennan holds an undergraduate degree in Biology from Bridgewater College in Virginia and he is board certified by the American Board of Foot and Ankle Surgery in foot surgery as well as the American Board of Podiatric Medicine. He is a fellow of both organizations as well.

Dr. Johnston is a podiatrist at a Tampa area hospital where she helps to teach and train podiatric residents. She holds an undergraduate degree in Biology with a minor in Psychology from Kentucky Wesleyan College in Owensboro, Kentucky. She is double board certified by the American Board of Foot and Ankle Surgery in foot and reconstructive rear foot and ankle surgery.

Together, the doctors coauthored the article "Underlying Synovial Sarcoma in a Patient with a History of CRPS: A Case Report," which was published in the *Journal of Foot and Ankle Surgery*. They also coauthored the children's book *The Footprint Hunt*.

INDEX

ABOUT CIDER MILL PRESS BOOK PUBLISHERS

Good ideas ripen with time. From seed to harvest, Cider Mill Press brings fine reading, information, and entertainment together between the covers of its creatively crafted books. Our Cider Mill bears fruit twice a year, publishing a new crop of titles each spring and fall.

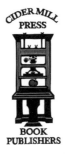

"Where Good Books Are Ready for Press"

**Visit us online at
cidermillpress.com
or write to us at
PO Box 454
12 Spring St.
Kennebunkport, Maine 04046**

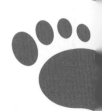

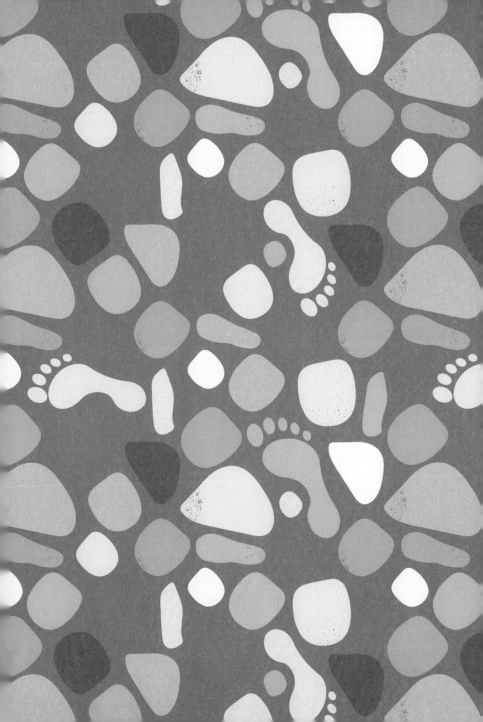

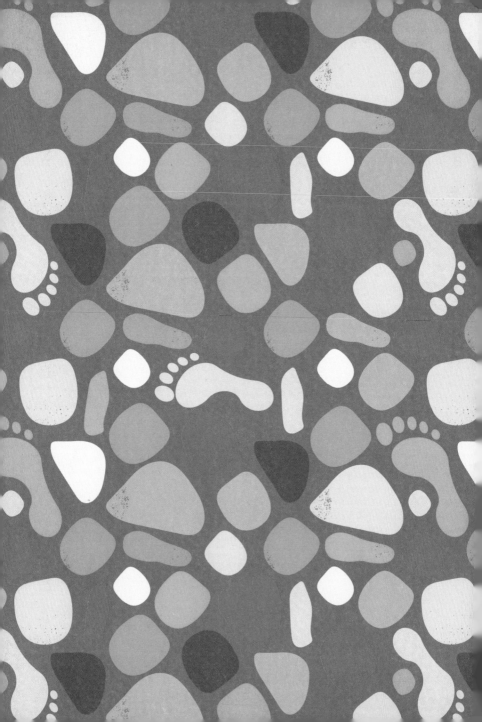